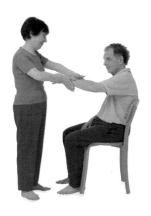

Health And Healing
The Natural Way

HANDS ON
HEALTH

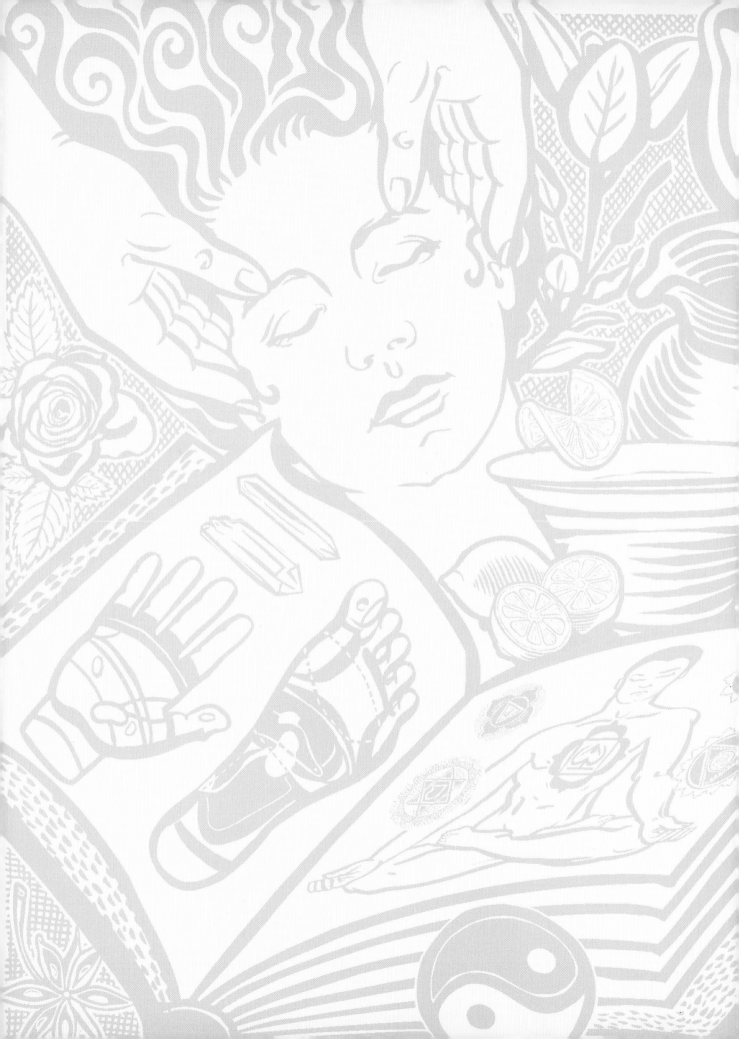

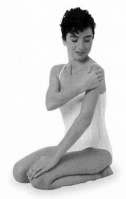

HEALTH AND HEALING
THE NATURAL WAY

HANDS ON
HEALTH

PUBLISHED BY

THE READER'S DIGEST ASSOCIATION, INC.

PLEASANTVILLE, NEW YORK / MONTREAL

A READER'S DIGEST BOOK
Produced by
Carroll & Brown Limited, London

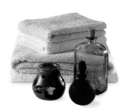

CARROLL & BROWN

Publishing Director Denis Kennedy
Art Director Chrissie Lloyd

Managing Editor Sandra Rigby
Managing Art Editor Tracy Timson
Project Coordinator Laura Price

Editor Jennifer Mussett
Art Editor Karen Sawyer
Designers Evie Loizides, Rachel Goldsmith,
Mercedes Pearson

Photographers Jules Selmes, David Murray

Production Wendy Rogers, Karen Kloot

Computer Management John Clifford, Paul Stradling

First English Edition Copyright © 1998
The Reader's Digest Association Limited,
11 Westferry Circus, Canary Wharf,
London E14 4HE

Printed in the United States of America
ISBN 0-7621-0146-6

The information in this book is for reference only;
it is not intended as a substitute for a doctor's diagnosis and care.
The editors urge anyone with continuing medical problems
or symptoms to consult a doctor.

CONSULTANTS

Charles Hunt, DO, MRO
School of Osteopathy, London

Graham Mercati, TCM
Massage consultant

CONTRIBUTORS

Bevis Nathan, MA, DO(Hons), MRO
*Consultant in alternative health,
osteopath, and osteopathy lecturer*
Maria Mercati, BA(Hons), ITEC, MTI, DS,
CERT. Tuina and Acupressure from Shanghai, China
*Consultant in massage therapies,
massage therapist, and writer*
Robin Kirk, MSc, ND, DO, MRO
*Consultant in manipulative therapies
and osteopath*
Jonathan Nunn, DO, MRO
*Consultant in energy rebalancing therapies,
osteopath, and healer*
Siobhan McGee, BA(Hons), TIDHA
*Consultant in aromatherapy
and aromatherapist*

FOR THE READER'S DIGEST

Series Editor Gayla Visalli

READER'S DIGEST GENERAL BOOKS, U.S.

Editor in Chief, U.S. General Books Christopher Cavanagh
Editorial Director, health & medicine Wayne Kalyn
Design Director, health & medicine Barbara Rietschel

READER'S DIGEST BOOKS & HOME ENTERTAINMENT, CANADA

Vice President and Editorial Director Deirdre Gilbert
Managing Editor Philomena Rutherford
Art Director John McGuffie

Address any comments about *Hands on Health* to
Editor in Chief, U.S. General Books, Pleasantville, NY 10570

HANDS ON HEALTH

More and more people today are choosing to take greater responsibility for their own health care, rather than relying on a doctor to step in with a cure when something goes wrong. We now recognize that we can influence our health by making improvements in lifestyle, for example, a better diet, more exercise, and reduced stress. People are also becoming increasingly aware that there are other healing methods—some of them new, others ancient—that can help prevent illness or be used as a complement to orthodox medicine.

The series *Health and Healing the Natural Way* will help you to make your own health choices by giving you clear, comprehensive, straightforward, and encouraging information and advice about methods of improving your health. The series explains the many different natural therapies that are now available, including aromatherapy, herbalism, acupressure, and a number of others, and the circumstances in which they may be of benefit when used in conjunction with conventional medicine.

The physical and emotional comfort provided by touch can help you stay healthy and feeling good about yourself. Furthermore, touch is recognized today as an important healing component in recovery from illness. Touch therapies can offer much-needed relief in a huge range of maladies. They can help realign muscular and skeletal imbalances, refresh the mind, stimulate the circulation and immune systems, and revitalize the body's energies. All touch therapies promote harmony by balancing the body, emotions, and mind. *HANDS ON HEALTH* offers you a survey of the wide range available and how to gain the most benefit from them. Some are based strictly on physical massage, while others have a spiritual root as well; some are vigorous and best reserved for the fully fit, while others are gentle enough for babies. No matter which touch therapy is most suited to your needs, it will help you relax and ease away the stresses of everyday life.

CONTENTS

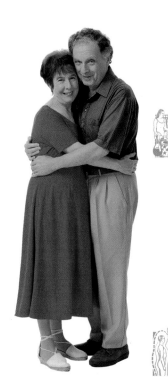

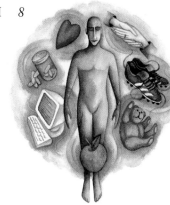

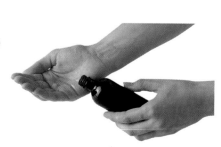

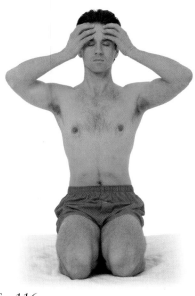

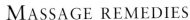

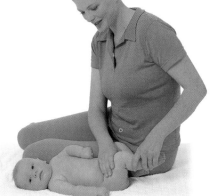

5 MASSAGE REMEDIES

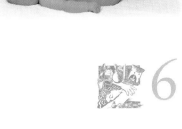

6 HEAL YOURSELF WITH TOUCH

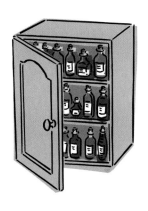

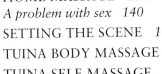

THE POWER OF TOUCH

One of the most natural and potent tools of health and healing, touch provides warmth, relaxation, and an inner feeling of well-being and peace of mind.

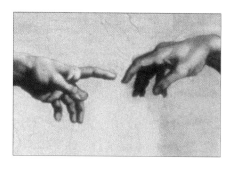

FEELING CONTACT
The sense of touch is an important and powerful means of communication, connecting individuals to the world around them and helping them feel secure, calm, and at ease.

BALANCING EXERCISES
Many touch therapies use stretches and exercises to enhance relaxation. This stretch is used in chiropractic to realign the backbone.

Touch therapies provide some of the crucial ingredients for good health, happiness, and relaxation, making you feel more confident, more in charge, and better able to live your life the way you want. Regular therapy sessions can bring about significant physical and mental changes, helping you to deal with emotional problems and cope more easily with life's ups and downs. Touch therapies are used regularly all over the world to provide support and relief for those who need them.

Touch can also be a profound expression of human affection, and it forms one of the most powerful tools of communication between two people. The need for physical contact is innate; the feeling of someone else touching us is naturally soothing, bringing a sense of calmness and comfort.

TOUCH FOR HEALTH AND HAPPINESS

There is a wide range of touch therapies, originating from all around the globe and founded on local traditions and knowledge. *HANDS ON HEALTH* looks at these therapies in three main groups: massage therapies, which deal with the physical benefits of massage; manipulative therapies, which include techniques to help improve the general functioning of the body; and energy rebalancing therapies, which aim to restore the balance of energy within an individual. Many of the latter originated in Asia and encompass philosophies that often use diet, exercise, and other approaches as well as touch to enhance an individual's health.

Most touch therapies operate on a holistic level; working with the whole person to promote balance, health, and harmony. Holistic philosophy links the physical body, mind, emotions, and spirit. Each affects and is affected by the others. For example, touch therapies can soothe muscles and relieve tensions in the body, which in turn enables the mind to relax and release emotional strains that have built up. Emotions can also affect the body; when the act of touch helps us to feel emotionally secure and relaxed, this eases our physical stresses and enhances our general health.

Holistic therapies aim to actively involve the individual, emphasizing the need for each person to take responsibility for his or her own health and take into account physical well-being, emotional makeup, belief systems, and lifestyle.

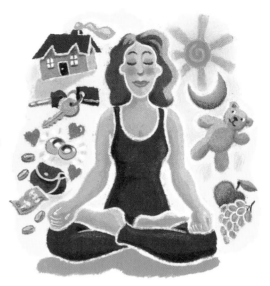

HOLISTIC THERAPIES
Holism is the concept that all parts of a person's life are inextricably linked, including work, health, relationships, family, and personal beliefs and goals.

TOUCH FOR FRIENDS AND FAMILY

Touch stimulates feelings of warmth, creating a sense of well-being and acceptance. The sensory experience of another person's hands is an instinctive comfort, making you feel happy and loved. Touching is the most sensuous and potent form of communication, and home massage can help you express affection for those close to you.

When first massaging a friend or family member, it is best to start slowly because many people are not used to being touched in this way. Society has long associated touch with the intimate relationship between a parent and child or between sexual partners. Touch therapies are an ideal way to break this barrier, allowing others to enter your touch circle. However, it is important that both the massage giver and receiver feel comfortable.

Massaging children and babies can be fun as well as good for their health. It can help them to develop, aiding both their physical and mental aptitudes. It might also be enjoyable to let them massage you, although their skills and patience will obviously be better if they are older. It can be very relaxing to let young children lie or sit on your back, but only if they are small—under seven years old—so they do not put a strain on your back.

REVITALIZING YOUR INNER SPIRIT

Many therapies use touch to fine-tune the spiritual balance. For the most part, these originated in the Orient and India and focus on unblocking energy channels and rebalancing universal energy, or qi (pronounced chee). Whether or not a patient fully understands the theory, the effect can be remarkable and has been known to help

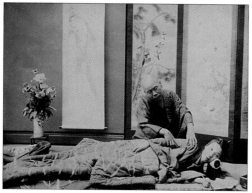

***GLOBAL TRADITION OF
TOUCH THERAPIES***
*From earliest times, touch
has been known to be a
natural and fundamental
healing tool. The Japanese
have been using massage in
the form of shiatsu and other
techniques for more than
two millennia.*

THE FIVE ELEMENTS
*Many touch therapies from
the Orient are based on the
five natural elements. Wood is
represented by the dragon, fire
by the phoenix, earth by the
ox, metal by the tiger, and
water by the snake.*

people with emotional problems, stress, and general
poor health, although perhaps its most marked result
is a surge of happiness and well-being. In recent years
many people in the West have taken up energy
rebalancing therapies and a more spiritual approach
to life. These approaches are becoming more accepted
as both alternative and complementary to Western
medicine and lifestyle, and many people have found
a spiritual balance through touch therapies.

There has been particular interest in the Eastern
therapies of shiatsu and Tuina. These are based on ancient systems
of living that aim to balance all the parts of human life, including
health, work, relaxation, and spiritual energy running through
meridians, or energy channels, within the body. The principles of yin
and yang—the presence of two opposite forces within every living
being—is central to these therapies, emphasizing the need for
balance and harmony in every individual.

The Five Elements—wood, fire, earth, metal, and water—are other
important components of these therapies. It is believed that they
should be balanced within a person, and a predominance of one
element means a deficit of another. A practitioner will consider the
balance of the Five Elements, using a patient's physical health and
emotional character as a basis for diagnosis. The rebalancing of the
whole person is then carried out through touch therapies that focus
on unblocking the 14 meridians that run down through the body,
each of which is linked to one of the Five Elements.

The framework of such approaches as polarity therapy is based on
the chakra system, which originated in India. The chakras are
believed to coordinate the flow of spiritual energy and are envisaged
as wheels that run in a line down the center of the body. The
flow of energy is dependent on both physical and psychological factors, such as fears, anxieties, and feelings of self-
esteem and acceptance. The aim is to open the chakras,
correcting the movement of energy to its natural optimum.
Some touch therapies like Reiki work on the principle that
many ailments are a physical manifestation of deeper
emotional and psychological problems; for example, back
problems may be caused by insecurity, and throat problems by
a need for expression. Such therapies aim to redress the entire
balance of an individual through self-realization, touch therapy
techniques, and lifestyle considerations.

MEETING YOUR TOUCH REQUIREMENTS

The 1990s saw a growing enthusiasm for the use of touch in health. The Royal College of Nursing in London found that massaging babies makes them significantly less likely to become ill and helps them grow stronger and faster. Babies denied touch will spend their energies worrying and feeling lonely, especially when their other senses remain undeveloped and they feel no other communication from the outside world. The Royal School of Midwives, also in London, has stressed the importance of touch during the first year of a baby's life. It has been realized that when babies emerge from the womb, where they have been in constant physical contact with their mothers, they feel the loss of this state of security and touch, particularly during the first six months of their lives. Touch therapies can provide consolation, helping babies to retain that feeling of safety and security. This need remains with each person throughout life, and touch therapies can offer adults a similar sense of reassurance.

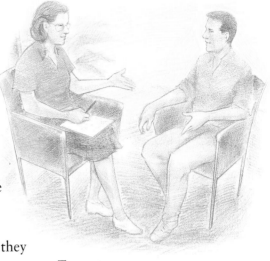

TALKING
A touch therapist will discuss your problems with you, whether they are physical ones or the emotinal stresses of everyday life.

STRESS RELIEF

Touch is an important tool for the relief of stress, easing tight muscles and relaxing the mind. Stress can build up in various parts of the body, leading to a number of problems, including back pain, stomach ulcers, irritable bowel syndrome, and heart conditions. All of these can be helped by touch therapies.

Touch therapists have identified particular areas of tension in the body and developed theories on what this tension can tell us about a person's psychological state. For example, the shoulders store emotional denial; the back holds the strains from anxiety and defense; and the pelvis area is affected by problems with sex, pleasure, and fear. There is an emphasis on getting back in touch with the natural instincts, listening to the needs of emotions and the body, and addressing any physical problems or contradictory feelings that might arise. It is often these difficulties that cause stress and lead to illness and a loss of vitality.

HOME MASSAGE
Learning to give and receive massage from friends and family can open the door to hours of relaxation and pleasure and deepen your relationships.

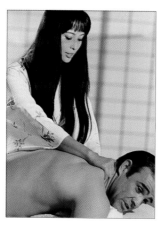

JAMES BOND
From the film You Only Live Twice, *this still shows James Bond (played by Sean Connery) enjoying the pleasures of a relaxing massage.*

EQUIPMENT
A number of items can be used to enhance touch therapies. These include aromatherapy massage oils, massage balls and rollers, skin brushes, and sponges.

Touch therapies have also become important in relieving the discomfort and distress associated with long-term illness. Studies in hospitals of patients suffering from chronic diseases such as cancer and AIDS have found that touch therapies can improve their condition as well as make them more comfortable. Reiki has had proven success in comforting patients with advanced cancer. A study of multiple sclerosis patients in Great Britain in the mid-1990s found that they had a positive reaction to reflexology: it reduced their symptoms, gave them more energy and a more positive outlook, and made them feel better in general.

DISCOVERING TOUCH THERAPIES

There are many types of touch therapy; each one employs a variety of techniques to tackle different health issues. Chapter 1 offers a comprehensive picture of what kinds of touch therapies are available. It includes a brief history of each approach and traces the development of different techniques from around the world.

Massage therapies are described in Chapter 2; they include Swedish massage, sports massage, and various massages from the Pacific islands, India, and Southeast Asia. Step-by-step instructions on the basic Swedish massage strokes and some Thai techniques are also included. The manipulative therapies—osteopathy, chiropractic, physiotherapy, metamorphic technique, and Rolfing— are covered in Chapter 3. These therapies employ joint movements, posture correction, deep-tissue work, and exercises to restore physical balance, flexibility, and range of movement in the body.

The energy rebalancing therapies are dealt with in Chapter 4. Most of these originated in the East, although some, such as reflexology, were developed in the West and have incorporated elements of Eastern energy theories. Spiritual principles involved in energy rebalancing are introduced along with the techniques.

Chapter 5 offers step-by-step instructions on massage methods that can be used at home to treat a number of common physical ailments and emotional problems. Setting a calm scene for a home massage helps to put both partners in a relaxed mood, and Chapter 6 is full of advice and ideas for creating an atmosphere conducive to a soothing session. It includes details on how to give a home massage, as well as information on aromatherapy oils and how to use them effectively. Throughout *HANDS ON HEALTH*, self-help features show how you can benefit from touch therapies at home.

WHAT CAN A TOUCH THERAPY DO FOR YOU?

Ranging from an invigorating Swedish massage to a spiritual Reiki session, touch therapies encompass a wealth of healing potential. They can help you cope with stress, depression, or grief, speed recovery from an injury or accident, or revitalize your inner energy and set you back on the path to health and happiness.

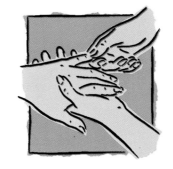

Q CAN TOUCH THERAPIES LESSEN ACHES AND PAINS?

There is a full range of touch therapies that can deal with physical problems or conditions. Manipulative approaches such as osteopathy and physiotherapy are now widely used to rectify physical complaints and aid recovery from injuries or surgery. A good massage can also revitalize a tired mind or exhausted body, helping you feel refreshed and ready for new challenges.

Q CAN TOUCH THERAPIES HELP ME WITH PERSONAL EMOTIONAL PROBLEMS?

Touch therapies can be used to deal with a range of emotional problems, including depression, stress, relationship difficulties, and insomnia. The physical relaxation and soothing effects induced by touch can be highly comforting, enabling sufferers to restore their balance and energy in order to resolve problems.

Q CAN TOUCH THERAPIES HELP MY IMMUNE SYSTEM?

By easing stress and tension, touch therapies play an important part in boosting the efficiency of your immune system, improving your body's natural ability to ward off illnesses. Certain touch therapies can also improve lymphatic drainage, thus helping to clean out the system and strengthen it.

Q HOW CAN TOUCH THERAPIES RELIEVE STRESS?

When touch therapies relax the body, tensions and stresses that have built up are naturally released, thus enabling the system to restore itself. We all suffer from stress and need time to relax properly and allow our bodies to recover. Touch therapies give us both physical and mental relief, helping us to regain a sense of calm and equilibrium.

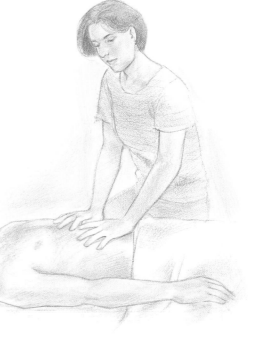

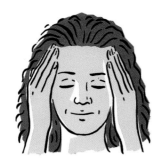

Q **WHAT IS MEANT BY SPIRITUAL ENERGY?**
Close your eyes, relax your body, and take a few deep breaths; you will feel good energy enter you and bad energy leave. Spiritual energy is believed to be naturally within you and all around you in the environment, and can be given to and received from other people. Energy rebalancing therapies aim to help you revitalize your spiritual levels, allowing you to tap into your intuition and understand life in a deeper and more profound way.

Q **CAN I IMPROVE MY RELATIONSHIPS WITH MASSAGE?**
Massaging your friends, family members, or partner can bring you closer together and give you an opportunity to talk over problems or grievances. Massaging babies and small children can be very good for their well-being, nurturing feelings of comfort, security, and love. Elderly relatives can also benefit greatly from touch, especially if they live alone and have little physical contact with others. Remember that everyone needs touch for the security, happiness, and health that it provides.

Q **HOW WILL I FEEL AFTER A TOUCH THERAPY?**
Following a touch therapy, you will experience feelings of deep relaxation, well-being, and contentment. Many people use this time to reflect on their lives from a positive and unstressed point of view. Touch therapies often entail an element of psychological and lifestyle readjustment, challenging existing patterns and fostering lifestyle changes to allow the recipients to live life more fully.

Q **CAN TOUCH THERAPIES HELP IN THE LONG TERM?**
Touch therapy can improve your health and general well-being, boosting your blood circulation, lymphatic drainage, and immune system, and helping to mend injuries. Stress relief and deep relaxation can revitalize you, enabling you to look beyond small problems and realize your own needs, abilities, and goals. The ultimate aim of most touch therapies is to act as preventative medicine, promoting long-term health and encouraging emotional and psychological understanding and happiness.

CHAPTER 1

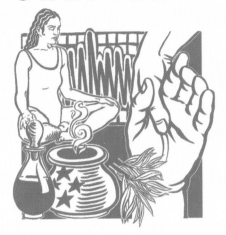

THE HEALING TOUCH

*The power of touch has been acknowledged
throughout history as one of our most effective and
instinctive healing forces. From the comforting
embrace of a parent to the soothing strokes of a
masseur, touch can help ease anxiety and tension and
restore inner balance in both body and mind.*

THE HISTORY OF TOUCH THERAPIES

Every culture worldwide has made use of the powerful healing qualities of touch. It has been highly valued for emotional comfort, pain relief, and spiritual healing.

Touch is one of the oldest and most instinctive forms of healing, an innate action to soothe and comfort those in need. There is evidence of touch healing throughout the recorded history of humankind, the oldest reflected in cave paintings from 15,000 years ago. The development of touch as a healing tool starts with the primitive instinct, displayed by both humans and animals, to offer comfort to another being who is vulnerable by providing physical contact—through cuddling, stroking, or holding, for example.

With humanity's increasing sophistication, touch therapy diversified into forms of faith healing, or spiritual healing, and more down-to-earth, massagelike rubbing. Over time, touch healing acquired complex explanations and interpretations, such as the spiritual concept of subtle energy transfer and the analysis of the anatomical mechanisms of the bones, joints, and muscles that lay the foundations for osteopathy. The development of modern medicine has brought a fuller understanding of the workings of the human body, and touch therapies have taken on a major role in health care, rehabilitation, and healing.

ANCIENT MASSAGE

Massage, the most widely practiced touch therapy, has been used for pain relief and relaxation for at least 5,000 years. It was the first and at one time the most important medical technique and is recognized today as a powerful, all-purpose therapeutic tool.

Ancient Chinese massage

The earliest reference to massage for healing comes from China, where there was a fairly sophisticated medical philosophy as early as 3000 BC. Chinese massage developed along-

---

TIMELINE OF TOUCH THERAPY

Comforting touch is an innate and natural response to pain, stress, and sadness. Since ancient times different cultures have built sophisticated touch techniques around the central tenets of touch healing.

c.15,000 BC
Cave paintings found in China show massage healing techniques in use before the development of known civilization.

c.3000 BC
Chinese medicine men formulated the acupressure system that is a major part of traditional Chinese medicine.

c.1800 BC
The first written references to touch therapies appeared in Indian texts. It is believed that touch therapies spread into India from the Orient.

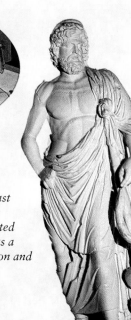

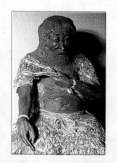

c.1000 BC
Massage spread from the East to ancient Greece beginning about 1000 BC. It was adopted by Asclepius the physician as a basic tool for the preservation and restoration of good health.

CATEGORIES OF TOUCH THERAPY

The three broad categories of touch therapy are massage, energy rebalancing, and manipulation. Each type is underpinned by a different theory—sometimes a whole philosophy—of health, illness, and healing. However, they all have one thing in common: the promotion of relaxation.

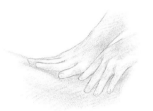

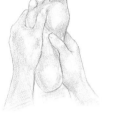

MASSAGE
This is the stimulation of blood flow by rubbing and stroking the skin. It can be deep or shallow.

ENERGY REBALANCING
Touch and pressure are used to balance the body's energies and release any blockages in the channels.

MANIPULATION
This corrects misalignments of the musculoskeletal system by manipulation, stretching, and exercise.

side acupuncture. Both recognize the importance of unblocked energy flow and have been used mainly for the maintenance of good health rather than the treatment of specific conditions. Modern Chinese massage, or Tuina (push-pull) is practiced widely in orthodox medical settings throughout China. From China, massage spread to India before 2000 BC, and the first writings about it date from around 1800 BC.

Shiatsu in Japan

Shiatsu, from Japanese words meaning finger pressure, combines aspects of Chinese medical philosophy and acupuncture with massage. At first called Anma, shiatsu is based on the concept of qi (pronounced chee), or energy flow, through the body via meridians, or channels. There are points along these meridians where qi is believed to accumulate. The points, called tsubos, correspond to acupuncture points in Chinese medicine. One goal of a shiatsu practitioner is to free trapped energy from these points.

Although shiatsu gained official recognition in Japan only in 1955, there are now more than 80,000 registered practitioners. It has subsequently become extremely popular in the West as well, especially for its relaxing and stress-relieving qualities.

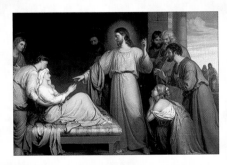

c.AD 30
The Christian gospels give 26 instances of Jesus healing by touch. Many religious leaders before and since are believed to have been blessed with the power to heal by touch.

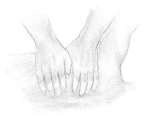

c.AD 500
Japanese touch therapies based on traditional Chinese medicine were developed to form Anma, which later grew into shiatsu.

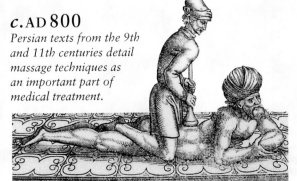

c.AD 800
Persian texts from the 9th and 11th centuries detail massage techniques as an important part of medical treatment.

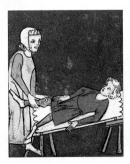

AD 800–1400
Although manipulation was used in the Middle Ages, it was often associated with magic and witchcraft.

Greek and Roman massage

Massage spread to ancient Greece from the East and was practiced for health maintenance along with exercise beginning about 1000 BC. It is described by Homer and subsequently by Hippocrates (the father of modern medicine) as part of the therapeutic regimen recommended for warriors. It is clear that Hippocrates used massage extensively in his treatments and understood some important massage principles. He also seems to have noticed the general healing effects of touch itself.

The Romans continued and expanded the Greek use of massage. It was used at the baths, along with various cleansing, stimulating, or relaxing oils, and was a respected medical therapeutic treatment in its own right. The physician Celsus wrote extensively on the application of massage for a great variety of ailments, and the writings of many other Greek and Roman figures, from physicians to philosophers, included lengthy sections on the importance of massage.

Egyptian healing

The Ebers Papyrus (1552 BC) is the oldest Egyptian medical text known. It contains a very sophisticated medical treatise on the use of medicines, including manual therapy. Before this time, Imhotep, a court architect during the 3rd dynasty (2700 BC), is recorded as possessing healing powers through the "laying on of hands." Some sources argue that the Greek god-physician Asclepius is somehow linked to the cult of Imhotep.

THE DECLINE AND REVIVAL OF MASSAGE

Although many Roman physicians and others living during the decline of the Roman Empire wrote favorably about massage, its popularity waned during the Middle Ages. It is not known why this happened, but one theory is that certain early Christian Romans abolished the baths because they had become places where sexual practices were more common than healing ones.

In Europe during the Middle Ages, art, science, education, and medical practices did not progress much and in some cases went backward. Massage and other traditional medicines became associated with magic or witchcraft, and folk healers who practiced them were often persecuted. Until the European Renaissance in the 14th and 15th centuries, there was much fear and ignorance about health matters and a withdrawal from care and attention for the physical body. However, Greek and Roman ideas and practices were preserved by the Arabic cultures, with massage described in prominent Persian medical texts written during the 9th and 11th centuries.

Massage was re-established in European medical practice during the 14th, 15th, and 16th centuries as a result of the renewed interest in sciences that came with the Renaissance. Advances in anatomy, physiology, and pathology informed massage practice and introduced increased sophistication.

In the early and middle 19th century, Per Henrik Ling, a Swedish physiologist and

1300–1600

The Renaissance revived the ideals of the ancient Greeks and Romans, including the physical enjoyment and pleasures of bathing and massage.

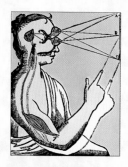

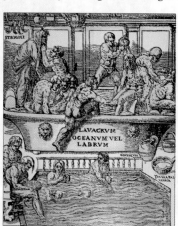

1600–1800

The Age of Reason saw the birth of modern science and medicine and separated the mind from the physical body.

1800–1900

Massage became recognized as a medical tool throughout northern Europe, particularly in Scandinavia and Germany.

1840–1900

The moral codes that were pervasive during the Victorian era discouraged nudity and touch. Touch therapies fell into disrepute, often because of associations with sex and prostitution.

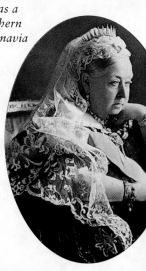

fencer, developed massage techniques into a more structured system. Ling's manipulating cure spread throughout Europe, Russia, and eventually North America and became the forerunner of both physical therapy and massage. The Dutch physician J. Mezger gave massage further scientific credibility by asserting that it was an essential aspect of rehabilitation. Mezger also popularized the French term *massage*.

Throughout Germany, Denmark, Norway, and Sweden in the latter half of the 19th century, massage was a commonplace and standard medical practice. In Britain, however, its reputation became tarnished by the growth of unscrupulous and corrupt massage institutes that advertised deceptively and offered inadequate training, producing incompetent practitioners. During this time many clinics gradually became centers of prostitution, or "massage parlors." The sorry state of the profession was formally reported in 1894 when a British Medical Association inquiry exposed the general lack of massage training and professionalism.

Furthermore, Victorian sexual prudery and religious puritanism tended to generate confusion about sensuality and sexuality, sadly culminating in an attitude of fear or disgust toward the flesh. Massage was seen as base, sordid, and even sinful. Although attitudes in the mainstream have changed, there still remains an ambivalence about touch and its link to sexual intimacy.

The spectacular advances in technological medicine throughout the 20th century lured

HIPPOCRATES

The Hippocratic system was based on rebalancing the body through exercise, diet control, and herbs. It incorporated some of the most vigorous manipulation techniques in the world for the treatment of soldiers and warriors. Some Eastern treatments still include similarly intense practices.

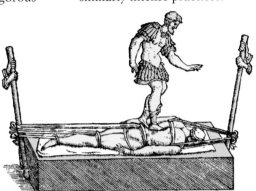

HIPPOCRATIC TECHNIQUE
Forceful traction and pressure were the main principles behind Hippocrates' vertebrae treatments, upon which many types of manipulation were formulated.

both medical and lay people away from massage and other forms of natural medicine. However, the considerable resurgence in touch therapies now evident is testimony to some of the failures of modern medicine to address the broader needs of the individual, especially the emotional needs and problems associated with care.

Despite its long history, touch is still poorly understood and remains underutilized as a healing skill. Used in the right way, touch improves trust, respect, and interpersonal communication. It enhances intimacy, induces relaxation, and feeds the silent hunger for touch that resides within us all.

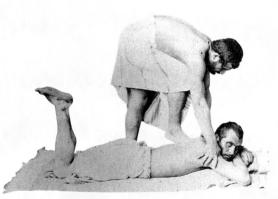

c.1870–1900
The 1870s saw a resurgence of interest in traditional therapies, and physicians, bonesetters, caregivers, and healers began to use natural therapies, including massage.

1914–1918
During the First World War nurses and other caregivers were trained in massage.

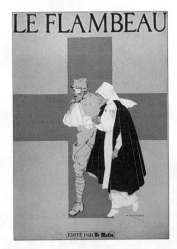

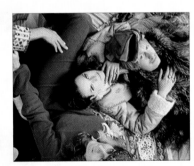

1960 ONWARD
The 1960s saw a rejection of social prudery. More emphasis was placed on natural and instinctive ways of living and healing, including a revival of touch therapies.

PHYSICAL BENEFITS

Touch therapies can leave you feeling vibrant, balanced, and relaxed. This is because they work at a level deeper than the skin, benefiting internal organs, blood circulation, and overall health.

The benefits of massage start with the skin itself, where an increase in blood supply and stimulation of the pores and tissues help keep it flexible, healthy, and young looking. Using oils along with massage also moisturizes the skin, keeping it supple and free from wrinkles. But touch therapies play a greater part in the body's general health as well, relieving problems in the central organs and revitalizing them.

RELIEVING MUSCLE TENSION
Perhaps the best known and most obvious effect of all hands-on therapies is the easing of muscle tension. This release is always accompanied by the mental relaxation associated with pain relief, which can last many days after treatment.

Muscles are the body's biggest users of energy and blood and have the greatest involvement in the activity of the nervous system. If they are in a state of tension, they sap a person's vitality. Muscle tension, can also mask severe fatigue through sheer nervous activity. Chronically tired patients often report extreme drowsiness and a pleasant lowering of intellectual focus directly after a deep massage, indicating that muscle tension has been released and underlying fatigue has been exposed. When arranging for a massage session, do not plan any challenging work immediately afterward: you might not feel in the mood to concentrate properly.

IMPROVING CIRCULATION
Patients receiving touch therapies frequently experience a warm glow directly after treatment, a physical sensation that may persist for many hours. During this time they may feel somewhat flushed and appear pinker in the face than usual. These warming effects are caused by a general improvement in the circulation of blood throughout the body. This is a normal and natural result, especially from those therapies that involve deep-tissue massage.

Blood needs to circulate at a regular speed, taking food and oxygen to all parts of the body and enabling them to function properly. If the blood circulation is sluggish, then some portions of the body will not get the food and oxygen they need. This occurs mainly in the hands and feet and leads to joint and skin problems. In extreme cases it may even cause paralysis.

LOWERING BLOOD PRESSURE
High blood pressure is associated with strokes and heart disease and is one of the most important signs of deteriorating health. While there is no hard evidence to date that touch therapies are able to lower a

---

MASSAGE AND YOUR SKIN

There are thousands of touch receptors just beneath the skin that enable you to feel the different pressures of touch. As sensations are received, messages are sent to the brain via the central nervous system. The brain processes the information and responds accordingly with muscle action, hormonal change, or an emotional response.

SENSING TOUCH
There are various touch receptors under the skin's surface.

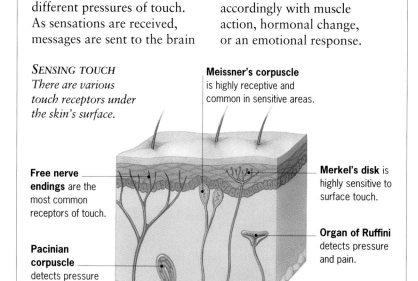

Meissner's corpuscle is highly receptive and common in sensitive areas.

Free nerve endings are the most common receptors of touch.

Pacinian corpuscle detects pressure on the skin.

Merkel's disk is highly sensitive to surface touch.

Organ of Ruffini detects pressure and pain.

OSTEOARTHRITIS

Osteoarthritis, also known as degenerative arthritis, is the most common type of the disease. It involves a wearing down of the cartilage on the joints, caused by continuous rubbing and usage. It can occur in middle age but is usually not serious until a person is well into old age, when it can cause problems with everyday tasks. Difficult to treat, osteoarthritis sufferers can benefit from careful massage, which can aid mobility of the joints and ease pain (see page 108). However, in more advanced stages of osteoarthritis, massage can be harmful and medical attention must be sought.

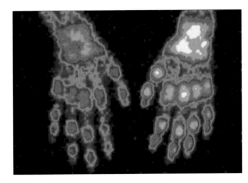

OSTEOARTHRITIS IN THE HANDS
This electroscan shows hands crippled with osteoarthritis. The brightness of the colors at the joints indicates the severity of the condition.

patient's blood pressure permanently, many studies have found that blood pressure tends to drop during massage as a result of the relaxation response. The reduction in tension produced by massage treatment is accompanied by a corresponding relaxation of the muscles in the blood vessel walls, which are responsible for increasing and decreasing blood pressure.

The extent to which touch can promote relaxation and better healing was revealed by an experiment at Ohio State University in the 1970s. Researchers fed large groups of rabbits high-cholesterol diets to determine what detrimental effects cholesterol might have on their blood vessels, particularly development of atherosclerosis, which causes heart attacks and strokes. The researchers were surprised to find that one group of rabbits developed 60 percent less atherosclerosis than the group as a whole, even though they had been eating exactly the same foods. Eventually they discovered that the healthier rabbits had been cared for by a certain technician who always picked them up, stroked them, and talked to them during the feeding routine. Almost disbelieving that the relationship factor could influence a bodily disease so tangibly, the researchers repeated the experiment, using, as before, the same diet for all the rabbits but this time designating that half of them regularly be picked up, stroked, and talked to. Again, the handled rabbits developed 60 percent less disease than the others. They concluded that touch played a significant role in helping the rabbits avoid illness.

EASING STIFF JOINTS

Stiffness in muscles and joints can be the result of simple strains, wear and tear from repetitive movements, old injuries, poor posture, or an area of the body compensating for a dysfunction in another area. Touch therapies can relieve these kinds of joint stiffness. Rhythmical moving of the joints stimulates the secretion of synovial fluid, thus lubricating them, and gentle manipulation of tight muscles relaxes tension, making movement easier and less painful.

Joint and muscle stiffness caused by osteoarthritis can also be relieved by touch therapies, but an inflamed joint should never be massaged directly. The areas surrounding it should be rubbed or kneaded instead.

PROMOTING HEALING

Healing from any illness involves the whole person. Illnesses don't get better; people do. Two things remain at the core of any person's ability to recover from ill health: first, having some sort of control over the course of the illness, and second, having a helpful and open relationship with a competent and caring physician or therapist (see page 33).

All touch therapies foster increased self-awareness and positive feedback about a patient's reactions to stress and illness. These effects are vital, especially for those people who have a poor

TOUCH FOR HEALTH
At a very simple level, touch therapies draw on the feelings of security and comfort provided by close physical contact with another person.

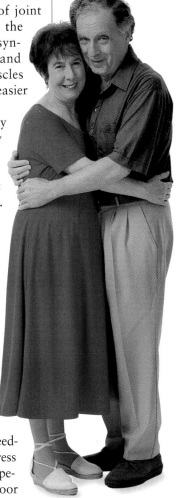

BENEFITS FOR THE BODY

Each touch therapy benefits health in different ways, which are broadly covered below. Some focus on lymphatic drainage, others on stiff joints, and some emphasize relaxation. Refer to the table on page 30 to find out which technique is most suitable for treating particular conditions.

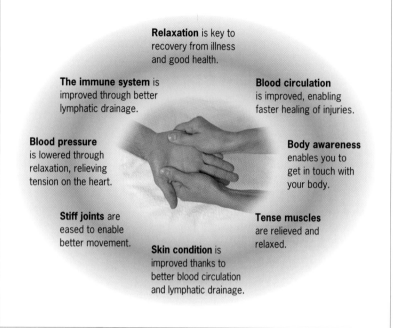

Relaxation is key to recovery from illness and good health.

The immune system is improved through better lymphatic drainage.

Blood circulation is improved, enabling faster healing of injuries.

Blood pressure is lowered through relaxation, relieving tension on the heart.

Body awareness enables you to get in touch with your body.

Stiff joints are eased to enable better movement.

Tense muscles are relieved and relaxed.

Skin condition is improved thanks to better blood circulation and lymphatic drainage.

Manipulative therapies promote healing by helping to integrate mechanical function of the joints and muscles. They also work by eliminating sources of pain, malfunction, and inflammation, so that the different systems of the body operate in their proper unified manner.

Energy-based therapies promote healing by increasing the flow of vital energy through diseased or dysfunctional tissues and by restoring balance and harmony to all the systems of the body. There is also a powerful feel-good factor involved in energy rebalancing, and this helps to revitalize a patient, encouraging a feeling of well-being, renewed vitality, and inner joy.

BOOSTING THE IMMUNE SYSTEM

The immune system is the body's internal disinfectant, attacking invading viruses and bacteria. The cells responsible for destroying hostile microorganisms are significantly less effective when a patient is under stress, so relaxation is an important factor in the efficient functioning of the system.

The immune system depends to a great extent on the lymphatic system, which collects the lymphatic fluid that cleanses the body's tissues and recirculates it via the blood. Without normal, easy flow of this lymphatic fluid, vital aspects of the immune system function poorly, and by-products of cellular biochemical reactions cannot be re-channeled or eliminated from the body. Poor lymphatic drainage creates a kind of stagnation in the tissues. Touch therapies, which stimulate healthy tissue-fluid movement, have long been credited with the ability to dramatically improve the functioning of lymphatic drainage.

understanding of the nature of their illness. Feedback from touch therapies can enable them to better understand their psychological and physical responses to being ill and encourage them to gauge the success of their coping behaviors more effectively. All these benefits enhance the patients' abilities to control their own bodies.

Massage-based therapies promote healing by encouraging deep relaxation, probably the single most effective healing strategy of all. Energy that has become locked in the muscles is liberated and can be used for healing and restoring full health.

INCREASING FLEXIBILITY

Touch therapies, particularly those that involve stretches and pressure techniques, can help patients become more keenly aware of their body—how it normally moves and feels, how flexible it is, and what its physical limitations are.

Touch therapies can provide the necessary tool for relaxing the restraining tensions in muscles and joints. Stretches and manipulative techniques have the effect of releasing restrictions in movement, increasing flexibility, and allowing the body to move in an unrestrained manner, thus enhancing posture and improving all-round health.

JOINT MOBILITY
Touch therapies aid joint mobility by stimulating the secretion of synovial fluid within the synovium, or synovial capsule. This lubricates the joint and eases movement.

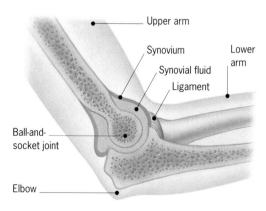

Upper arm

Synovium

Lower arm

Synovial fluid

Ligament

Ball-and-socket joint

Elbow

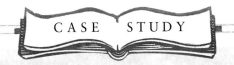

A Backache Sufferer

Many people with back pain believe they must have done something strenuous to injure themselves, but cannot remember any particularly traumatic event. However, backache can often be caused by built-up stress and lack of regular physical activity. Touch therapists can help relieve the pain and encourage patients to alter their lifestyles.

Peter has been a taxi driver for all of his working life. He is 58 years old and married to Rachel, a part-time nursery school teacher. Over the past 10 years the volume of traffic has grown so much that Peter has found each journey takes a lot longer and his income has dropped. For some time now, to compensate for diminishing returns, he has been working a longer day, neglecting his morning exercise routine, and spending less time in the evening with his wife and family. Peter has noticed a low backache developing over the past six months. One recent afternoon, while lifting a passenger's bags, he felt a sudden severe lower back pain, which forced him to leave work early. A friend recommended an osteopath.

WHAT SHOULD PETER DO?

Peter visited the osteopath, who diagnosed a simple muscle strain in the lumbar spine and indicated that it should heal quickly. But Peter has been lifting passengers' bags easily all his life, so the underlying problem is muscle weakness, which can be remedied only by daily stretching and toning exercises.

Peter needs to face the fact that he is getting older and that overwork and strains are likely to manifest themselves more readily in his body. He and Rachel should discuss whether he needs to continue working such long hours or if an alternative income can be found so that he can go back to his normal hours. He also needs to take time to relax and restore his family life.

Action Plan

SPOUSE
Get together with Rachel and discuss whatever needs airing. Share concerns, no matter how apparently trivial.

STRESS
Initially, get more sleep, as fatigue clouds judgment. Work out finances and lifestyle priorities carefully. Make a plan to avoid worrying about small pressures.

EXERCISE
Perform gentle stretching and back-strengthening exercises daily before work. Take up a weekend activity, perhaps with the family.

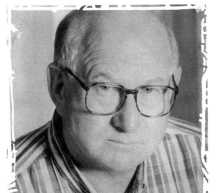

EXERCISE
Regular exercise is vital for sedentary workers in order to prevent undue muscle weakening.

SPOUSE
Relationships can begin to suffer when habitual overwork leads to poor communication and mistaken assumptions.

STRESS
Long-term overwork with insufficient rest causes fatigue and tension, which can lead to dysfunction in any muscle group and potential muscle breakdown.

HOW THINGS TURNED OUT FOR PETER

After a few months of regular osteopathic visits, Peter's back was better. He found it easy to resume his exercise routine, which is counteracting the weakening effects of prolonged sitting. He and Rachel joined a badminton club, and they talk together more often in order to uncover any worries. They decided that Peter should cut his work hours and developed a plan for sharing household chores so that Rachel can return to work full-time.

COULD A TOUCH THERAPY HELP YOU?

Touch therapies can help with all sorts of problems and symptoms, improving your overall health and well-being. This questionnaire will enable you to measure your own condition and give you an indication of the range of problems that hands-on therapies can address.

Consider each question carefully and write down the number given next to each question. When you have finished, total the score and compare it with the advice for that score at the bottom of the page to find out whether you are in need of a good, relaxing massage.

QUESTIONS

Do you ever have difficulty relaxing?

yes	score 3
no	score 0

Do you often have trouble sleeping?

yes	score 3
no	score 0

Do you feel tired and lacking in energy?

yes	score 3
no	score 0

Do you need any of the following to get you through the day?

alcohol	score 2
tobacco	score 3
caffeine	score 2
painkillers	score 4

Have you had any major problems in the past 6 months?

legal problems	score 4
problems at work	score 3
redundancy	score 6
retirement	score 3

Do you suffer often from any of the following?

migraine	score 4
minor illness	score 3
stiff joints	score 3
backache	score 6

Do you ever need sleeping pills?

yes	score 4
no	score 0

Have you had any family problems?

yes	score 3
no	score 0

Do you suffer from digestion problems?

yes	score 3
no	score 0

Do you need to improve your blood circulation and general health?

yes	score 2
no	score 0

Do you often get caught up in everyday things and forget to enjoy life?

yes	score 3
no	score 0

Do you have an ongoing illness or condition that is difficult to treat?

yes	score 5
no	score 0

Has anybody close to you died within the past year?

spouse or partner	score 12
close family	score 10
close friend	score 6

Have you had any of the following relationship changes in the past year?

marriage	score 3
separation	score 6
divorce	score 10

Have you had a major upheaval in the past 6 months?

moved home	score 5
change of job	score 4
become a parent	score 2

Do you worry too much?

yes	score 3
no	score 0

Do you constantly feel rushed?

yes	score 4
no	score 0

Would you like to feel more relaxed?

yes	score 2
no	score 0

Have you had any of the following in the past 6 months?

major illness	score 6
operation	score 6
major accident	score 6
major injury	score 6

Do you have any of the following continual stress factors?

a baby or toddler	score 3
young children	score 5
teenage child or children	score 3

Have you experienced any of the following problems in the past 6 months?

loss of interest in sex	score 4
sex problems	score 6
lack of sexual fulfillment	score 4

SCORE

0-30

If you scored under 20, you have a healthy and unstressed life. A touch therapy will help you to stay balanced and enhance your relaxation. If you scored between 21 and 30, the idea of a relaxing massage is most likely quite appealing. You are probably dealing with a few stressful problems and your health could be better. Try a relaxing massage, or if you have any specific health problems, refer to the table on page 30 to find a touch therapy that can help treat your problem.

31-60

If you scored between 31 and 60, you are probably having a difficult and challenging time at the moment. Your health is not as good as it could be, and you have a high level of stress in your life. A touch therapy is important for your emotional and physical health. It will help you to relax and calm down, enabling you to cope and recover properly through this difficult period. Particular problems can be improved by specific therapies; the table on page 30 can help you find the touch therapy you need.

Over 61

If you scored more than 61, you could benefit greatly from a relaxing touch therapy. It could help with physical problems (see the table on page 30) and provide general relaxation and stress relief, giving you a breather from everyday worries and time to replenish your energy. Many touch therapists provide additional help by offering advice on how to relax or simply by being there to talk to. Some therapists also offer counseling services or psychological help.

MENTAL BENEFITS

Every day we face emotional stresses that build up in our muscles and tissues, causing tension and discomfort. Touch therapies can soothe these strains and relax the mind.

It is not possible to be mentally anxious and physically relaxed at the same time. The body responds to thoughts and feelings with muscle tension and glandular secretions. The more that thoughts or feelings cause worry or hurry, the more tense the muscles become and the body chemistry changes inappropriately. In reality, there is no difference between mental and physical tension and no difference between mental and physical relaxation. Treatments such as touch therapies, which promote physical relaxation, also enhance mental relaxation.

WHY RELAXATION IS IMPORTANT

The human body is built to move, and so in this sense the muscle, bone, and joint systems are the primary systems of the body. These tissues operate most efficiently when periods of exertion are followed by periods of rest. Overdoing either of these activities can lead to problems. Deprived of regular exertion, the musculoskeletal system remains understimulated, and deprived of rest, it cannot replenish itself.

A continuously stressful or exhausting lifestyle will push the body beyond its boundaries, sometimes for long periods of time. Deep relaxation will allow the body's own systems to rebalance themselves and is more likely to promote healing than any other single activity. This is why all physicians agree that the healing powers of sleep cannot be matched by any medicines.

DID YOU KNOW?

The ancient Greeks believed that the physical body was intrinsically linked to the mind, the emotions, and even the personality. Our use of the word "melancholy" stems from the Greek notion that depression was caused by black bile, or *melankholia*.

Relaxation and self-awareness

Before real relaxation can take place, a person must become aware of the sensations felt in his or her body when it is at rest. Many people think they are relaxing when, in fact, they are merely distracting themselves by reading or watching television, for example. Distraction allows large groups of muscles to remain rigid without the person being aware of this fact.

One of the most efficient ways of bringing the body to awareness is to receive touch, and making patients more aware of their bodies and posture is one of the primary goals of manual therapy. Many manual

BENEFITS FOR THE MIND

The mental benefits of touch therapies differ from one type to another but can have profound and long-lasting effects. Relaxation of the mind is a primary benefit of all touch therapies, helping you to forget everyday worries and feel happy—a sure and sound route to good overall health.

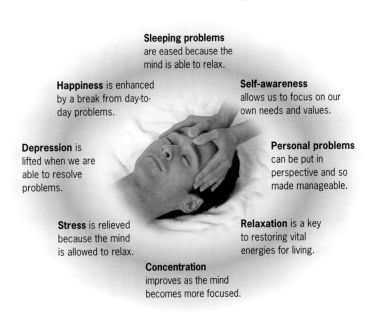

Sleeping problems are eased because the mind is able to relax.

Happiness is enhanced by a break from day-to-day problems.

Self-awareness allows us to focus on our own needs and values.

Depression is lifted when we are able to resolve problems.

Personal problems can be put in perspective and so made manageable.

Stress is relieved because the mind is allowed to relax.

Relaxation is a key to restoring vital energies for living.

Concentration improves as the mind becomes more focused.

Stretch for energy
Simple stretching can be done virtually anywhere to relieve muscle tension and boost energy levels.

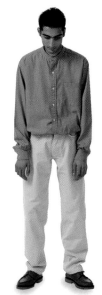

DEPRESSED SLOUCH
Slouching can make you feel down and lacking in vital energy.

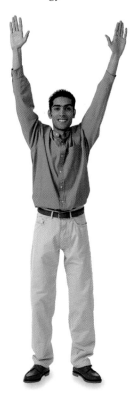

HAPPY STRETCH
Stretching releases tensions and stimulates vitality and energy.

RELAXING THE BRAINWAVES

Brainwaves are electronic pulses that run through the brain, transmitting messages and solving problems. When we are awake, beta waves dominate the brain. These are short, quick waves that help us through everyday situations. When we are asleep, the longer delta waves dominate. In between the two stages, when we are drowsy and deeply relaxed, alpha waves occur. This alpha state can be achieved through massage, helping us to draw closer to sleepiness.

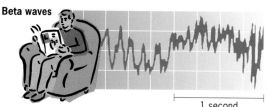

Beta waves

1 second

STATE OF BEING AWAKE
Beta waves are dominant when we are awake and our mental processes are functioning. The waves are short and close together, enabling us to think quickly.

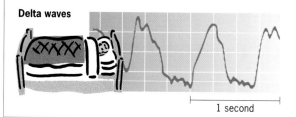

Alpha waves

1 second

STATE OF RELAXATION
Alpha waves occur just before falling asleep, during or right after a massage or during meditation. The waves are slower and longer, easing us into a sleeplike state.

Delta waves

1 second

STATE OF SLEEP
Delta waves, which are large and slow, predominate when we fall asleep. They allow the brain to relax completely, and they foster healing and proper rest.

touch therapists encourage this by suggesting that patients concentrate on the sensation of the treatment in order to become reawakened to their bodies and to the feelings, memories, and thoughts that are stored as physical sensations.

RELIEVING INSOMNIA
Insomnia is a complex condition, but the basic elements are straightforward. It is important to remember that different people need different amounts of sleep. For example, it is generally accepted that with increasing age, less sleep seems necessary. Anxiety about insomnia only adds to the problem; usually the worst consequence is worry about being tired and not functioning well with insufficient sleep.

Recipients of touch therapies often remark that after a treatment they feel extraordinarily tired and they sleep longer and more deeply. This may be a feature of every session if the person is chronically tired. The main reason is that touch thera-pies expose underlying fatigue by helping to reduce the stress-coping hormones that keep people going under pressure. This is part of the relaxation response: relaxing massage and exercise will induce tiredness in sleep-deprived subjects.

Sleep is often prevented by the presence of tension, which is a physical and mental phenomenon. Touch therapies are very effective at reducing muscle tension, whether by physical stretching and deep massage or by the promotion of a balanced energy flow. Together with the encouragement of adequate and balanced blood circulation, these effects enhance the body's ability to sleep.

Some people have fidgety bodies; they twitch in various areas when they are trying to sleep. This is caused by the buildup of pockets of tension within the nervous system, which discharge themselves when the demand for regular movement is lifted at bedtime. Touch therapy can provide channels for releasing this energy naturally and can prevent its periodic buildup.

RELIEVING DEPRESSION AND GRIEF

Depression is constraint placed upon self-expression, while grief is an emotion characterized by sorrow. A depressed person may be emotionally inhibited, whereas a grieving person may be very expressive.

Although distinct from each other, grief and depression are often thought of together. Both are normal, as long as they are appropriate to a situation and are temporary. Grief or depression following the death of someone close is a natural reaction.

An emotion is a bodily process, not just a mental recognition of a feeling. Generally, the more that people are aware of and express their grief appropriately, the more the grieving process is turned into personal growth rather than just a sense of loss. Touch therapies provide a caring forum for the grieving person and, through physical contact, can often allow the release of pent-up feelings that need an outlet.

RELIEF OF STRESS AND ANXIETY

The alleviation of stress is one of the most beneficial aspects of touch therapy. Stress and tension are nearly equivalent words and can mean almost anything that causes a mental or emotional feeling of unease. Anxiety and depression are forms of stress, but so are such other experiences as feeling embarrassed, frustrated, rushed, under pressure, and of course, in pain. Most people experience at least a little stress and anxiety every day, which is natural and harmless unless it becomes too much to manage and the body does not recover properly.

Another aspect of stress is a kind of mental and bodily confusion created when emotions are felt but not expressed, for fear of upset, anger, or embarrassment. The feelings are provoked by the "fight or flight" reaction—a primitive and powerful self-preservation reflex—but the expression of such feelings is generally discouraged by civilized societies. The body, having been set up to respond in an emotionally expressive way, is in effect prevented from doing so by the mind. The result is internal conflict, which can remain unresolved.

IMPROVING CONCENTRATION

True concentration is a mental habit of focusing the mind and intensifying specific mental acts of attention. It is enhanced when distraction by other subjects is minimal and when the body's needs do not unduly impinge upon the mind. Much of the theory of some touch therapies is devoted to exploring the ways in which treatment soothes unnecessary nervous activity. Nervous commotion in patients who have pain or discomfort or are out of balance ceaselessly bombards the brain with neurological noise—nerve information concerning bodily problems that require attention. Touch therapies can improve concentration by dealing with these internal bodily needs and promoting full physical and mental relaxation.

HOW TOUCH IS REGISTERED IN THE BRAIN

When you feel touch, the message is sent through the nervous system to the brain cortex where specific regions relate to the different parts of the body. The more sensitive the area to touch, the greater the size of the part of the brain that responds to it—for example, the hands, feet, face and mouth have the greatest sensitivity to touch and have a correspondingly large touch center in the brain.

TOUCH SENSITIVITY
This woman has been illustrated with her nonsexual body parts drawn in scale to their touch sensitivity. Her hands, lips, and feet are drawn largest, as they are some of the most sensitive parts of the body.

Improving your concentration

When our minds are tense or stressed, we cannot concentrate properly. Here are a few easy methods for boosting your concentration.

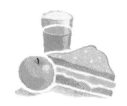

ENERGIZING SNACKS
Foods high in complex carbohydrates provide your body with fuel.

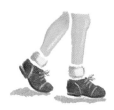

STRESS-FREE WALKS
Exercise frees the mind of mental work and improves blood flow.

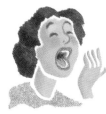

INVIGORATING YAWNS
We yawn to take more oxygen into our system and stimulate vitality.

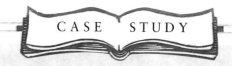

An Anxious Student

Many people who have physical aches and pains are actually suffering from anxiety and fatigue—a powerful combination, notorious for producing muscular discomfort. A patient might think such pain is evidence that a part of the body is severely malfunctioning, thus generating further anxiety and a vicious cycle of stress and more pain.

Mary is a 22-year-old university student majoring in marine biology. Two weeks before her final exams, a mild but persistent ache in her left shoulder, which she had had for a month or so, suddenly became unbearable, shooting up her neck and into the side of her head and culminating in a splitting headache whenever she tried to study for more than an hour at a time. The more she tried to work, the worse the pain became. She decided to go swimming before her evening study session, but this seemed to make matters worse. Her doctor diagnosed stress and prescribed painkillers, but when the painkillers failed to have any effect, Mary doubted the doctor's diagnosis and feared a more serious illness.

WHAT SHOULD MARY DO?

The student counseling service recommended regular massage to reduce tension. A masseuse confirmed the diagnosis by demonstrating, during a deep massage, that the condition was tension related. Mary admitted to her habit of studying with her head bowed over her books, a position that demands a lot from postural muscles. She also told the masseuse that she had been allowing herself only five hours of sleep a night for the preceding four weeks. She has been fretful and unable to relax, causing problems with her boyfriend and adding to her distress. Mary needs to become aware of her unhealthy habits, particularly with respect to posture, tension, and lack of sleep.

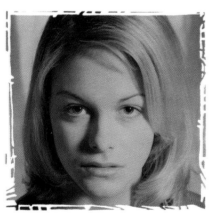

STRESS
Prolonged stress can be a direct cause of muscle tension and pain.

TIME MANAGEMENT
Failing to balance the different elements in your life can lead to health problems.

EXERCISE
Exercise involving exertion when already fatigued may prove counterproductive. Relaxation practice is often more appropriate.

Action Plan

STRESS
Stop the buildup of stress and tension by adopting good posture, stretching frequently, and taking regular relaxation breaks.

TIME MANAGEMENT
Break off at set times for massage, meals, sleep, relaxation training, and even a little recreation. Eat and sleep regularly.

EXERCISE
Take a brisk walk once or twice a day for at least 20 minutes. This measure can help relax the mind and body, easing tensions and aiding concentration.

HOW THINGS TURNED OUT FOR MARY

Mary started walking twice a day and made an effort to stop work for a few seconds several times an hour to stretch and relax into her chair, gently pulling her head upward and backward and dropping her shoulders. She continued to have massages through the examination period, finding them highly valuable. Mary also grew more self-aware and learned to recognize tension as it develops, thus becoming more self-reliant.

TYPES OF THERAPY

Each type of touch therapy has a unique approach and uses different techniques to relieve tension buildup in the body. It can be helpful to understand and even try out a number of them.

Because all touch therapies offer a variety of different techniques, for symptoms ranging from chronic arthritis to everyday stress, it is important to be well informed about them. Many people try out a few different approaches to find the most appropriate therapy and the right practitioner—one who makes them feel comfortable. Professional training standards and certification requirements for many of the therapies have greatly reduced the number of poorly trained practitioners, but care must still be taken when choosing a therapist.

MANIPULATIVE THERAPIES

These take an essentially mechanical approach to solving bodily problems. They involve using the hands in a variety of diagnostic and therapeutic methods, which vary not only among different manipulative disciplines but also among practitioners within the same discipline. The most well-known manipulative therapies are chiropractic, osteopathy, and manipulative physiotherapy.

Although manipulative therapists describe themselves as treating structural misalignments in general, it is true to say that they lay an emphasis on the muscular system first and foremost. The dysfunction most commonly seen by manipulative therapists is muscle tightness, or hypertonia. This condition interferes with proper joint functioning, feels uncomfortable, leads to fatigue, and disturbs effective overall bodily movement, thus leading to further stress and other physical problems.

Manipulative therapies emphasize careful palpation, or gentle squeezing, of the soft tissues to locate areas that may be showing increased strain or imbalance, which could result in more serious problems if unchecked. They also stress the need to identify what has happened or is happening in the patient's life to bring about such problems. A practitioner will discuss with a patient possible ways of changing the way he or she moves, works, plays, stands, sits, or lies down, in order to correct problems and prevent them from recurring.

Because all parts of the body relate to all other parts physiologically, each of these relationships can affect the rest of the body and mind if it becomes dysfunctional. When all of these connections are proper and balanced, they constitute a harmonious whole. A manipulative therapist works on the structure and function of the body with this ideal in mind.

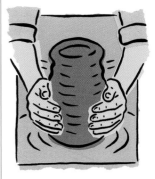

IMPROVING YOUR TOUCH

Pottery and other clay work can help your hands develop sensitivity. The smallest pressures can transform a ball of clay into a lovely pot or vase, and misplaced, insensitive pressure can turn it back into a misshapen lump. When you work with a ball of clay, first feel it between your fingertips to determine its softness and density.

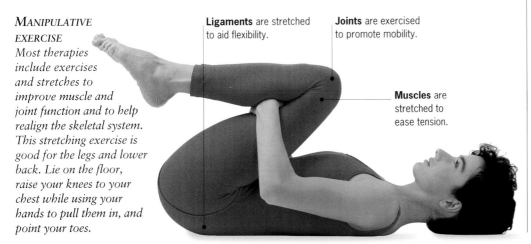

MANIPULATIVE EXERCISE
Most therapies include exercises and stretches to improve muscle and joint function and to help realign the skeletal system. This stretching exercise is good for the legs and lower back. Lie on the floor, raise your knees to your chest while using your hands to pull them in, and point your toes.

Ligaments are stretched to aid flexibility.

Joints are exercised to promote mobility.

Muscles are stretched to ease tension.

29

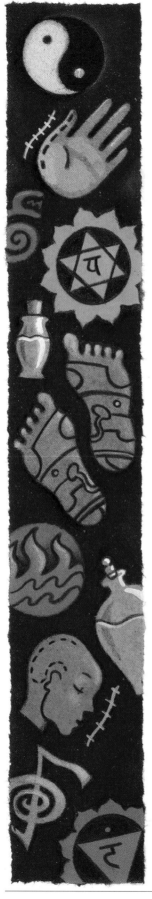

HOW TO CHOOSE A THERAPY

There are so many different types of touch therapy that it can be difficult to choose which is the right one for your condition or complaint. The table below summarizes many of the touch therapies available in North America. If you are interested in a particular therapy, simply look up the relevant page to find out more details.

THERAPY	DESCRIPTION OF THERAPY	WHAT IT IS GOOD FOR
Swedish massage page 40	Soft tissue and muscles are massaged for stress relief and relaxation. Often used with aromatherapy.	Relaxation, stress relief, stress-related disorders
Manual lymphatic drainage, page 43	Through massage of the lymph nodes, improves the lymphatic system, which cleans the body.	Poor circulation and problems with the immune system
Indian head massage page 51	The head, neck, and shoulders are massaged with oils. Good for sinus, hair, and skin conditions.	Relaxation, hair and scalp care, stimulating and energizing
Thai massage page 52	The pulling and stretching of the body. Excellent for relaxation, flexibility, and feeling good.	Relaxation, flexibility, poor circulation
Hawaiian massage page 53	Based on a deep spiritual intuition, this massage emphasizes relaxation and peace of mind.	Depression, low self-esteem, insomnia
Osteopathy page 62	The skeleton is realigned through stretches, thrusts, and manipulation. Good for back problems.	Recovery from injury or surgery, joint problems, backache
CranioSacral therapy page 66	Subtle pressure is applied to the skull to rebalance the central nervous system.	Skull disorders, birthing problems
Chiropractic page 68	Aims at realigning the spine to balance the central nervous system.	Recovery from accidents or surgery, joint problems
Physiotherapy page 70	A range of techniques are used, including heat, ultrasound, and hydrotherapy.	Muscular pains and strains, recovery from injury
Metamorphic technique page 74	This is based on careful massage of the feet to resolve problems encountered in the womb.	Relaxation, depression, confusion
Rolfing page 76	The deeper layers of the soft tissues that connect the muscles and bones are pummeled.	Relaxation, stress-related disorders, depression
Tuina page 80	Acupressure points are pressed to rebalance the flow of universal energy through the body.	Fatigue, lack of energy, depression
Reflexology page 84	Pressure is applied to parts of the feet to rebalance energy and heal problems in the rest of the body.	General health problems and feeling of imbalance
Applied kinesiology page 86	Asks questions and tests muscle reactions to help uncover allergies and other problems.	Specific psychological problems, finding allergies
Educational kinesiology page 88	Helps the brain to function properly through simple exercises that foster learning.	Poor concentration, poor learning skills
Shiatsu page 90	The body's energy system is powerfully rebalanced through pressure points. Good for all-round vitality.	Relaxation, lack of energy, confusion, stress
Jin Shin page 94	The hands are placed on energy centers to clear the energy channels. Good for self-understanding.	Emotional problems, stress, chronic illness
Reiki page 96	Universal energy is channeled through the healer to enhance spiritual and physical health.	Lack of energy, anxiety, confusion
Polarity therapy page 100	Massage, diet, exercise, and counseling are used to harmonize positive and negative forces.	General poor health, feeling of imbalance, and lack of harmony

MASSAGE THERAPIES

Massage is essentially a nontechnological practice that has in recent years acquired a somewhat more scientific standing. It is a profoundly human art, essentially healing in itself, and at its most basic, it requires no specific training. It derives from the instinctive and natural caregiving act of touching another person with a moving hand. A mother rubbing a child's sore arm to make it better is such an act. Parents who often stroke their babies and young children rarely do so consciously; theirs is an innate and automatic action.

Human beings communicate not just with spoken language but also through gesture and touch. Touch can often communicate most effectively where words have failed. With massage, however, the communicative aspect of touch is on a different level from that of instinctive actions because of the infantlike passivity of the recipient and the one-way nature of the active massage.

Mother-infant touch

Recipients of massage probably have not been touched in this way since infancy, when their mothers hugged, stroked, cuddled, rocked, and held them for a large proportion of time. The significance of these actions is not merely that recipients of massage may become transported to an infantile state. Mother-infant touch has been shown necessary for the physical, psychological, and social development of an infant. Touch used on an adult in this context is therefore capable of promoting and nourishing natural and basic self-healing qualities.

ENERGY-BASED THERAPIES

The fundamental concept upon which all energy-based therapies depend is that of the subtle body. This is a kind of nonvisible, energetic counterpart of the physical body, upon which the physical body depends both for vitality and organization. There are many variations on this theory, some of which are discussed in Chapter 4.

The doctrine of the subtle body, or subtle energy, is common to all religious traditions and ancient systems of philosophy. However, because it is not based on a rational foundation, it has been largely disregarded by modern Western society.

Healing based on spiritual theories predates modern medicine by more than three

TOUCH AND BABIES

A 1987 study examined whether touch could affect the development of 40 premature babies while they were being kept in incubators. Half the babies were massaged for 15 minutes, three times a day. Those receiving massage averaged 47 percent more weight gain than the control group.

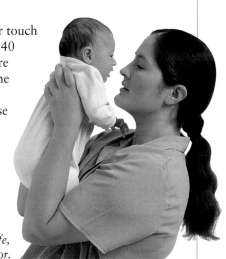

A MOTHER'S TOUCH
Touch is believed to be particularly important during early infancy, because in the first few months of life, it is the most mature sensory receptor.

millennia. Energy-based therapies work on the concept that subtle energy should flow around the body in a highly organized, specific way, providing vitality and order to the physical body. Disruptions to the harmonious flow of energy may be caused by excessive or insufficient energy, energy blocks, or disorganized energy, either at specific sites or as a broader theme.

The cause may be located at the energetic level or at an emotional or mental level. Once the energy flow is out of balance, a blockage in one area can exacerbate a problem in another, and a self-maintaining cycle is established. An energy rebalancing therapy reintegrates healthy energy flow.

BIODYNAMICS
Many spiritual therapies are based on the concept that our behavior should reflect the rhythmic patterns and energies of nature and the universe. This 15th-century Spanish star chart was used by healers to predict the healing energies and health of an individual from the position of the stars.

THE BALANCE OF MIND AND BODY

Relaxing the stresses on both body and mind, touch therapies harmonize the whole person, helping to restore inner balance and inspire self-awareness and self-fulfillment.

HOLISM
Holistic therapists view each patient as a whole, taking into consideration all the different aspects that make up a person. It is common for such a therapist to ask questions about personal relationships, work or social life, and emotional troubles.

The philosophy behind most touch therapies is that of holism, a term that is used by many health care practitioners but is often misunderstood by the lay person. It is an attitude toward healing, not a particular therapy. The word *holism* comes from "whole": a holistic practitioner tries to see a patient's problems in the context of a wider picture. This may involve looking at the relationships between different parts of the body, between the body and emotions, and between the patient and his or her partner, family, and work.

Most physical problems are connected in some way to these other areas. Naturally, practitioners cannot be expected to have

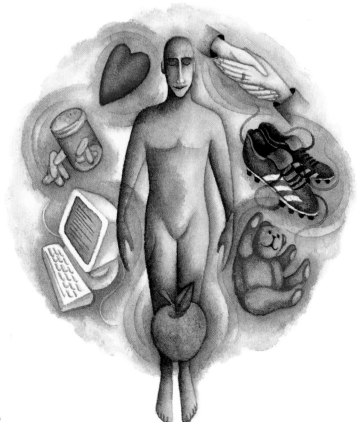

influence over all of them and must choose where their sphere of expertise begins and ends while realizing where additional help may be needed. No one can be a masseuse, osteopath, polarity therapist, general practitioner, and faith healer all in one, but every holistic practitioner has a duty to try to view a patient's problems as a sign that all is not well with the person as a whole and consider which aspect is best aided. For example, it may be unwise to prescribe medication for a patient whose symptoms are caused by stress at work. It might be more effective to suggest ways that the patient might achieve a measure of control over the working environment and methods of dealing with adverse reactions to stress.

Holism acknowledges that mental factors often play a significant part in the process of becoming unwell and in getting well again. The ancient Greek philosopher Plato stated that the medicine of his day paid too much attention to the body and not enough to the soul. More than 2,000 years later the same criticism is still leveled at the medical profession, and by no means do all natural therapists display a holistic viewpoint.

The aim of holistic therapies is to balance a person so that the vital energies of the emotions, the body, the mind, and the spirit can be mutually beneficial to each other rather than contradictory. Touch therapies are uniquely positioned to work toward this goal. Touching is, in normal human life, usually associated with expressing intimate aspects of relationships and as such is emotionally laden. There is often a profound psychological effect involved in touch therapy, which probably contributes in a major way to its healing powers. When this mind-body connection is respected and explored by both practitioner and patient, touch therapy can be a genuinely holistic tool that will promote all-round healing.

TOUCH THERAPIES THAT EXPLORE EMOTIONS

Understanding the link between emotions and physical health has led many touch therapists to include some sort of psychological dimension in their practice. This could be an informal chat about problems or a more structured psychotherapy session that attempts to analyze deeper issues.

In addition to polarity therapy, the metamorphic technique, and Jin Shin—all covered later in this book—there are some touch therapies that work specifically on deeper emotional responses. One of these, watsu (water shiatsu) is an emotionally stimulating treatment that focuses on resolving deep emotional trauma. The practitioner supports the patient in a pool while massaging him or her under the water. Emotional release is encouraged and is greeted with a calm and nonjudgmental acceptance.

Looyenwork, developed by Ted Looyen, a psychotherapist in California, attempts to change psychological patterns and resolve emotional troubles through massage and postural changes. The practitioner reads a client's psychological makeup from posture and the tension in muscles and joints. Through recognizing and relieving tensions, belief patterns can be challenged and problems resolved. Increased self-esteem, confidence, and relaxation are common results.

Zero balancing was founded in the United States by Dr. Fritz Smith, an osteopath and acupuncturist. It aims to clear the energy flows within the body, which can become clogged with either physical or emotional problems. A patient is put into a deep meditative state as the practitioner gets into a "dialogue" with the patient's energy fields.

RELATIONSHIP BETWEEN PRACTITIONER AND PATIENT

It is possible to divide the causes of healing into two categories: the effects of a particular treatment and the effects of the relationship between practitioner and patient. In practice, however, these two merge imperceptibly. In the case of touch therapies, the situations are much more intertwined than usual. Because touching is used in everyday life to express intimate aspects of interpersonal relationships, touch therapy, being physically intimate, is inherently a kind of close relationship itself. The quality of this connection is a strong element in therapy and the healing response.

In the sections on mental and physical benefits on pages 25–27, the effects of treatment are described as if they were independent of the practitioner. In reality, however, a practitioner who provides information, support, care, guidance, and companionship in addition to treatment is usually more effective than one who merely diagnoses, treats, and instructs.

The importance of the rapport between patient and practitioner is often underestimated. It is no accident that many patients try several practitioners until they find one with whom they get along well. Whether the practitioner is a massage therapist or an osteopath may turn out to be less important than whether or not the relationship formed is enjoyable, trusting, and confidence-inspiring. Finding the kind of trust that you need is often a very personal judgment, and it might be necessary to reconsider a recommendation from a friend: a therapist who is good for your friend may not be so well attuned to your problems. The connection between a practitioner and a patient can be healing in itself because mental and emotional processes play such a significant part in self-healing.

THE PATIENT-PRACTITIONER RELATIONSHIP

Finding the right touch therapist is crucial to a successful outcome. In some cases this decision can be more important than which therapy is chosen.

▶ *Trust is an essential ingredient in the relationship, enabling a patient not just to disclose sensitive information but also to relax more.*

▶ *A patient must have confidence in the practitioner's competence.*

▶ *Support is essential; a patient should feel that the practitioner can share the burden of his or her problems.*

▶ *A patient should feel that the practitioner has made a connection and is able to understand and help with problems.*

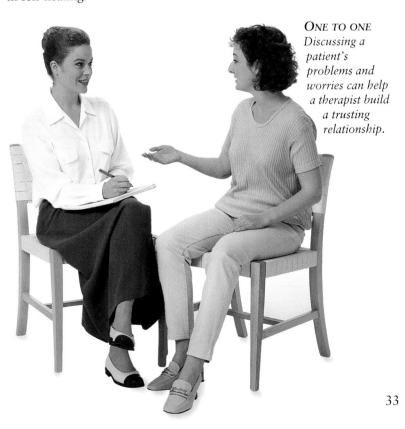

ONE TO ONE
Discussing a patient's problems and worries can help a therapist build a trusting relationship.

The Massage Therapist

Combining the skills of massage with anatomical knowledge and personal care, massage therapists can deal with a wide range of problems. They are often called upon to soothe and relax patients before and after surgery or other medical treatment.

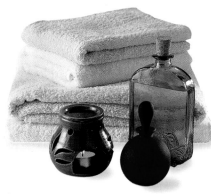

AROMATHERAPY
Many massage therapists have found that aromatherapy is a powerful tool for enhancing relaxation and aiding massage treatment.

What does a massage therapist do?

The therapeutic masseuse, or massage therapist, is trained to give a general-purpose, whole-body massage that is tailored to the individual needs of the client. The massage therapist therefore takes into account age, sex, body type, general health, energy levels, and areas of stiffness and sensitivity, in addition to any particular areas of dysfunction that might need particular attention.

The patients who benefit most from therapeutic massage are those with stress-related problems. The reason for this is also the reason that massage is successful as a therapy in

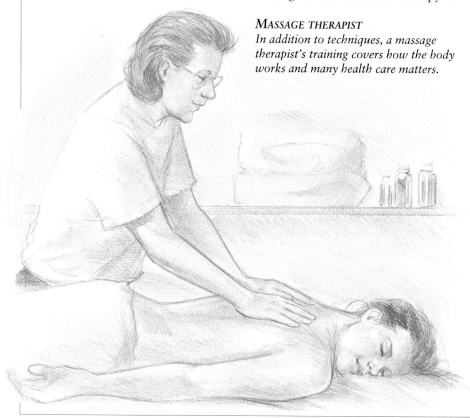

MASSAGE THERAPIST
In addition to techniques, a massage therapist's training covers how the body works and many health care matters.

general: it is a physical and emotional treatment at the same time, so the relaxation response is both physical and psychological. There is no cutoff between mind and body when it comes to slowing down.

The most obvious effects of stress are tight, unyielding, and achy muscles. Muscles in this state are probably more effectively loosened by massage and deep relaxation than by any other therapy, and this is why the massage therapist sees so many people with muscular disorders.

What training do you need to become a massage therapist?

A registered therapist holds a diploma from a recognized massage training institute. Training varies enormously from place to place because massage, by and large, is not regulated by any one institute or organization. In some jurisdictions it is not regulated at all. Most professional associations require members to have at least 500 hours of training at an accredited school; others require between 2,200 and 3,000 hours of training. Some British universities offer degree courses in therapeutic massage.

Most therapists are trained to understand both the physiological and psychological effects of massage and to know how to apply a wide range of styles and techniques, depending on the patient's problems. This enables them to adjust a massage treatment according to a patient's specific needs, both emotional and physical.

PREPARATION FOR MASSAGE

Most Swedish massage therapists combine massage with a sauna, steam bath, or soak in a hot tub. A sauna is a small, wood-lined room dry-heated to high temperatures; a steam bath consists of a tiled room filled with steam; and a hot tub has circulating jets of hot water. All serve to heat the body—relaxing muscles and encouraging the skin to sweat and expel dirt. Fifteen to 30 minutes in a sauna, steam bath, or hot tub will leave your skin warm, cleansed, and supple, ready for a thorough massage.

What symptoms can it help?
These range from very specific problems, such as tennis elbow, calf-muscle strain, fibrositis, and some kinds of back pain, to the effects of stress, anxiety, and emotional problems. The essence of therapeutic massage is to achieve deep relaxation of the whole body, which promotes self-healing in general. Any particular area of concern is then addressed specifically, usually following a full-body massage to revitalize blood circulation and relax the whole person.

Patients with structural injuries may be referred to a massage therapist by a doctor, osteopath, or chiropractor prior to further treatment. This is done to soothe the tissue and stretch out the fibers of any damaged muscles. It also improves blood circulation prior to osteopathic manipulation.

Who should not have a massage?
The abdomen, legs, and feet should not be massaged during the first three months of pregnancy. If you have a fever, a fracture, an infectious disease, swelling, skin inflammation, osteoporosis, thrombosis, varicose veins, large areas of bruising, severe back pain, cancer, or extreme fatigue, ask your doctor if you are a suitable candidate for a massage. With your doctor's advice, the therapist might modify the treatment in some way or avoid certain areas.

A qualified massage therapist is trained not only to decide what kind of approach may be of use but also to assess when a patient is unsuitable for massage and should be referred to another practitioner. Make sure that you tell a practitioner about any conditions you have or have recently recovered from. They may not seem relevant to you but could alert the massage therapist to areas that need treating with particular care.

What do doctors think?
The attitude of most doctors toward therapeutic massage is very positive. This is partly because such treatment is seen not as an alternative to orthodox medicine but rather as genuinely complementary to it, and it sometimes leads to improved health when other efforts have failed.

General practitioners find massage therapists especially useful for patients who have persistent aches and pains for which no medical disorder has been found; for the elderly who need physical contact for emotional reasons as well as to help keep their joint and muscle systems mobile; and for patients who are unhappy, lonely, anxious, or unable to relax. For this latter group massage usually provides a genuinely relaxing and therapeutic experience.

What happens in a session?
A massage therapist will take your case history, asking you questions about your reason for visiting. The practitioner will need to know about your medical history in outline and your current health in greater detail and will explain what he or she intends to do. You may also be asked about any work or emotional problems that you are experiencing and how they may be affecting your health: undue stress or anxiety, for example, could be causing trouble.

You will probably have to undress—clothes encumber most massage processes—although some people do prefer to remain partially clothed. The therapist will use towels, however, to cover those parts of your body that are not being massaged at any given time.

AFTER TOUCH THERAPY

A warm bath with a few drops of soothing essential oils is the perfect way to relax after a massage. Try a few drops of jasmine, lavender, or other oil that promotes calmness. Make sure that you won't be disturbed, and turn the lights down low or light a few candles. Soft music can enhance a relaxing atmosphere, although some people prefer silence after a massage in order to clear their minds completely, use the peace to restore their inner balance, or reflect on their lives and any problems or difficulties.

SKIN CARE
Massaging moisturizing cream or oil into your skin will help keep it smooth and flexible.

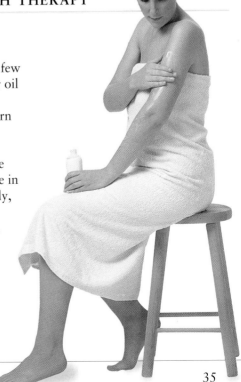

Spiritual touch

Throughout history touch has been recognized for its spiritual qualities. Faith healing, or the laying on of hands, employs the spiritual power of touch to restore health and well-being.

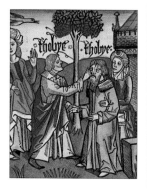

MEDIEVAL HEALING
During the Middle Ages the health of the body was often connected with spiritual servitude or witchcraft, and religious healers were often called upon to cure the sick.

ROYAL TOUCH
In medieval times, when doctors were scarce, royalty was believed to have the power to cure through touch, in particular, the "King's evil," a painful disease of the lymph glands also known as scrofula. This engraving depicts Charles II of France in the act of healing a sufferer.

Touch as a means of healing is a very old practice. When used in the context of a spiritual or religious belief system, touch is often called faith healing, or the laying on of hands. The term *faith* in this context refers to a mystical or religious belief in a higher order, as opposed to faith in a practitioner or method of health care.

FAITH HEALING

Faith in a healer who is drawing on a spiritual or divine power can be of two kinds: first, faith in the person who is conducting the healing, and second, faith in one's own spiritual belief that things not yet known will be revealed or that events not yet apparent will occur.

In the former, the patient's belief that the practitioner is capable of healing sets off a variety of completely natural inborn healing mechanisms. These are based on the individual's inner certitude that he or she is going to get better. This is not merely a kind of inner knowledge but one of emotional self-persuasion. Many people have experienced this same effect after consultation with a good medical practitioner. They feel better because they have been reassured about their condition and have become convinced of their practitioner's ability and competence. Talking about a favorite doctor or healer, patients will often say, "I have faith in him." This translates roughly as "I know he can help me" and forms the basis for the placebo effect, in which patients do get better because they believe they will.

History of faith healing

The history of spiritual faith healing is one aspect of the history of religion. It has long been believed that representatives of the divine, whether Christian ministers or Sufi saints, have been given special dispensation to heal by a supernatural power. Therefore, early examples of the laying on of hands fall largely within a framework either of religion or of magic, which is itself sometimes considered a kind of primitive religion.

The Christian gospels list 26 individual healings and 27 group healings by Jesus, and 9 multiple healings by his apostles. Jesus emphasized that his healing work was a channeling of God's love, and almost without exception, spiritual, or faith, healers describe their healing work as involving love or compassion. However, descriptions of faith healing may also refer more explicitly to healing energy. Such energy is said to emanate from a divine source if the basis of the healing is spiritual.

Illness as evil

The idea that illness is associated with evil is a very old one. Since ancient times many people have believed that illnesses are caused by gods angered by sins or by curses from spirits or people, either as deserved or undeserved punishment. Nowadays, some see bacteria and viruses as evil, invading us from all angles. We suffer from an attack of arthritis; we fight the battle against cancer. The language of medicine is littered with value-laden and military metaphors. It is almost as if we are innocent bystanders, assaulted by malevolent entities and in need of a knight in shining armor to aid our recovery and return us to complete health.

Indeed, it is still customary for doctors to be endowed by society with great power and social status because of their special knowledge and skills. It is in this power that patients put their faith, intensifying the possibility of getting better. More often than not, simple faith initiates healing from within.

THERAPEUTIC TOUCH

Therapeutic Touch is a modern version of faith healing, and though it may seem like a general term, it is increasingly being used to denote a particular technique that heals by channeling life energies from healer to patient. Unlike faith healing, Therapeutic Touch upon first examination appears to be independent of any belief in a divine or religious system, by either the healer or the patient. However, the theory of subtle energy, the basis of this healing method, is rooted in ancient religious philosophies. The healers who first recognized and developed the art of healing through touch were all profoundly religious people. Furthermore, and to its great credit, Therapeutic Touch encourages the development of spiritual values and beneficial self-care practices in the healers themselves, encouraging them to know themselves and get in touch with their own spirituality in order to help others.

Origins of Therapeutic Touch

The practice of Therapeutic Touch was founded by Dolores Krieger, a professor of nursing at New York University. It is quite natural that this healing technique should have arisen out of a nursing setting because nurses have always used touch as an expression of caring and compassion.

Krieger deserves much credit for helping establish not just a conceptual foundation but also an ethical basis for Therapeutic Touch through her insistence that the main prerequisite for learning the art is a sincere desire to help others, combined with a willingness to engage in honest self-reflection.

How it works

Essentially, Therapeutic Touch relies on the recognition that human beings have energy fields, associated with their physical bodies, that organize and give life to bodily processes. Krieger uses the Sanskrit term *prana* to describe this vital energy.

TESTING THE HEALING POWER

At the University of London in the 1980s, a series of controlled experiments were carried out to discover if there really was any basis for belief in spiritual healing. Dr. David Hodges and Dr. Tony Scofield, two lecturers in physiology, set up a scientific experiment: They left cress seeds in salt water overnight to make them effectively "sick," and then asked a spiritual healer to "heal" them. The seeds were divided into two groups, a control group and a pile that was given to the healer. He held the seeds in his hands and directed spiritual healing energy onto them for a few minutes. Both groups of seeds were then laid on wet tissue paper, and their growth was monitored. The results were that the seeds treated by the spiritual healer grew faster than the control group, suggesting that some form of energizing had taken place.

Healthy people appear to have an excess of prana. This is evidenced by their considerable capacity to avoid illness and disorder and an ability to call upon vast inner resources of energy when necessary. People who are obviously healthy are often described as vital or vigorous—a reference to an abundance of energy. Conversely, ill people seem to have insufficient life energy. They are constantly tired and unable to stay healthy. This can lead to a downward spiral and an inability to deal with problems.

Therapeutic Touch involves the transfer of vital energy from healer to patient, using the hands to direct the flow. The process can also be seen as a state of mutual resonance between the energy fields of the two participants, both of whom are in a constant state of flux with ever-changing energy.

According to the theories of the Indian system on which most energy rebalancing approaches are based, the vital energy within a person flows around the body through centers known as chakras. These are vortices of concentrated and organized energy, from which energy courses throughout the body into all tissues and organs. The chakras link the spirit, body, and mind with the universal flow of energy to harmonize the whole being. Each chakra controls a deeper level of self-realization, which helps a person reach a perfect state of fulfillment. In Therapeutic Touch, energy received by the patient is used to augment the inherent healing process, which involves a

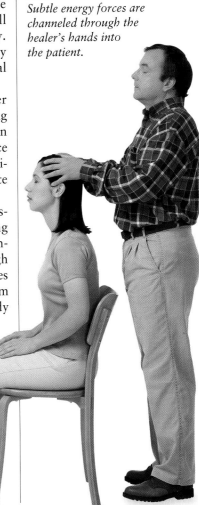

THERAPEUTIC TOUCH
Subtle energy forces are channeled through the healer's hands into the patient.

RELEASE YOUR SPIRIT

To achieve better control over your spiritual energy, try one or all of the following practices.

▶ *Practice meditation and reflection exercises.*

▶ *Contemplate your special place in the universe.*

▶ *Learn to accept yourself and others.*

▶ *To the best of your ability, try not to hurt any living creature.*

▶ *Try to help others and share your spiritual joy.*

rebalancing of energy by correcting any deficiencies or excesses or unblocking the flow where it has been stopped.

Therapeutic Touch requires that the healer become centered and meditative, with a deep intention both to direct energy with compassion and to remain detached enough not to influence the patient with his or her personal emotional energy. Some believe that in order to act as a vessel for spiritual healing energy, a person needs to be relatively free from personal troubles.

Training and practitioners

Dolores Krieger maintains that the capacity for Therapeutic Touch is inherent in all human beings and can be learned by "any physically healthy person who is strongly motivated to help ill people." She insists, however, that students should study themselves and their motivations carefully and recognize a desire to be respected, especially for their healing skills and faith in the spirit. The importance laid on self-realization and self-respect is a central tenet of the theory.

According to Krieger, all people can train their hands to become sensitive to the human energy field, and once they have acquired this ability, they can learn how to provide Therapeutic Touch. To get a sense of this energy field, hold your hands in prayer position, palms nearly touching; move them two inches apart and then return to the original position. Repeat the sequence twice, separating your hands four inches, then six. Finally, move your hands eight inches apart and pause every two inches as you bring them together. Hold them nearly touching for a full minute, concentrating on what you sense. You may feel heat, cold, pulsating, tingling, or another sensation that is a cue to your own energetic state.

In North America, Therapeutic Touch is taught in many nursing schools, and in the U.S. it has become popular as part of mainstream nursing practice. Although the method has remained predominantly within the nursing profession, it has also been taught to thousands of nonprofessionals.

Conventional opinion and research

Conventional opinion is divided on Therapeutic Touch. Some people are skeptical because the results are difficult to prove by scientific methods. Others have doubts because one widely publicized experiment by a youngster seemed to dispute the therapy's efficacy. Proponents, however, question the methodology of her experiment and point to the thousands that this practice has helped. So far, studies indicate that it can increase hemoglobin levels (the oxygen-carrying compound in blood), induce physiological relaxation, decrease anxiety, relieve pain, lower blood pressure, reduce stress, and accelerate wound healing.

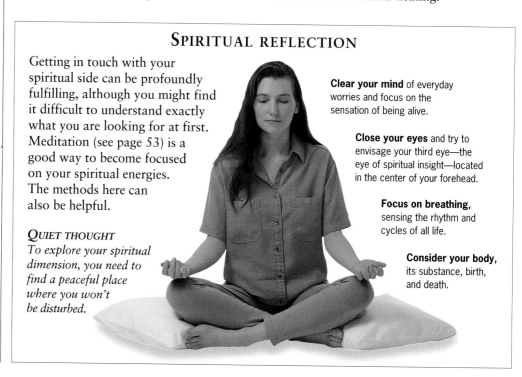

SPIRITUAL REFLECTION

Getting in touch with your spiritual side can be profoundly fulfilling, although you might find it difficult to understand exactly what you are looking for at first. Meditation (see page 53) is a good way to become focused on your spiritual energies. The methods here can also be helpful.

QUIET THOUGHT
To explore your spiritual dimension, you need to find a peaceful place where you won't be disturbed.

Clear your mind of everyday worries and focus on the sensation of being alive.

Close your eyes and try to envisage your third eye—the eye of spiritual insight—located in the center of your forehead.

Focus on breathing, sensing the rhythm and cycles of all life.

Consider your body, its substance, birth, and death.

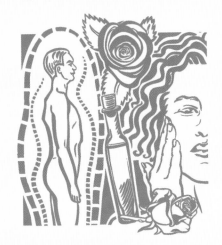

CHAPTER 2

MASSAGE THERAPIES

*Throughout history people in virtually every culture
around the world have harnessed the power of massage.
Western massage techniques seek primarily to provide
pain relief and general relaxation, whereas massage
treatments from the East focus on the mind-body
relationship and a more holistic health therapy.*

TYPES OF WESTERN MASSAGE

Western massage, based primarily on the Swedish system developed in the 19th century, focuses on relaxing muscles, improving circulation, and increasing mobility.

Most Western massage therapies are based on the Swedish techniques that were first formulated in the early 19th century. Many variations and special approaches have been developed for different conditions or situations; among them are remedial massage for muscular problems and sports massage for athletic conditioning and injuries. Aromatherapy massage combines Swedish manipulations with natural plant oils to enhance general health and well-being, as well as to treat specific conditions and illnesses.

SWEDISH MASSAGE

Although rooted in the remote past, modern Western massage is based almost entirely on a system devised by the Swedish physiologist Per Henrik Ling (1776–1839). Healing massage was not new to Europe in Ling's day; it is known to have been part of accepted medical practice in 16th-century France.

Ambroise Paré (1509-1590), personal physician to the French royal family, was a great believer in its therapeutic powers, and he is credited with having treated Mary, Queen of Scots with massage.

It was not until Ling, however, that massage became popular in its own right throughout the Western world. In 1813 a college was opened in Stockholm offering Ling's system as part of the curriculum. Its popularity spread rapidly and widely throughout Europe and North America during the 19th century.

However, in the early 20th century, especially after the First World War, the popularity of massage slumped, to a large degree because of the unfortunate comparison with the activities that took place in so-called massage parlors.

Since the 1960s there has been a major resurgence of Swedish massage, and it is now firmly established as a keystone of the relaxation and beauty industries. Its popularity has risen alongside increasing affluence, which has given more people the opportunity to improve their health through relaxation and stress relief.

Swedish massage techniques

There are three basic techniques: effleurage, or stroking; petrissage, or kneading; and tapotement, also known as percussion or tapping. The French names reflect the fact that French was the principal international language in Ling's day. Using these three methods, pressure and friction of varying intensities can be applied to the soft tissues of the entire body. In earlier times therapists used talcum powder to lubricate their hands during massage. Nowadays, massage oil is more commonly employed, often mixed

---

MASSAGE AND BEAUTY

Massage has long been known for its cosmetic benefits and beauty enhancement. From the ancient Romans to today's Hollywood stars, many have used it to refresh the skin and help keep the body looking and feeling young. The healthy glow that follows massage stems from the increased flow of blood to the surface of the skin. Relaxation is another bonus: a relaxed person looks healthier and more attractive.

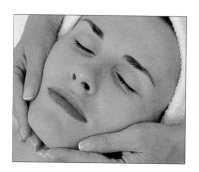

BEAUTY MASSAGE
Many beauty treatments include an all-over relaxing massage to improve skin condition.

HOW AROMATHERAPY WORKS

Aromatherapy oils affect you in one of two ways: chemically, through the bloodstream, or as a process in the brain. In the bloodstream, the active constituents in the oils affect the body in ways similar to those of herbal medicines—by altering chemical makeup and hormonal levels. As a brain process, scent stimulates certain feelings and hormonal reactions.

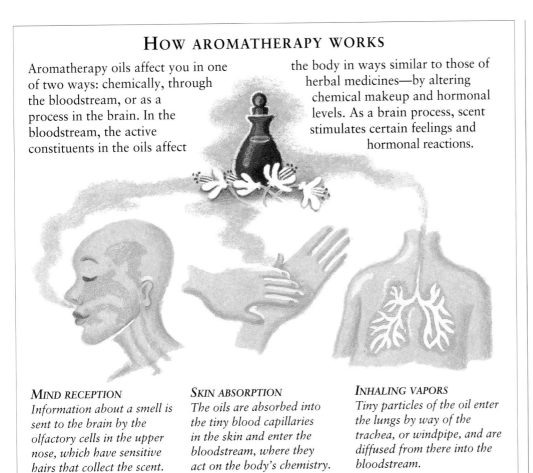

MIND RECEPTION
Information about a smell is sent to the brain by the olfactory cells in the upper nose, which have sensitive hairs that collect the scent.

SKIN ABSORPTION
The oils are absorbed into the tiny blood capillaries in the skin and enter the bloodstream, where they act on the body's chemistry.

INHALING VAPORS
Tiny particles of the oil enter the lungs by way of the trachea, or windpipe, and are diffused from there into the bloodstream.

HOW TO USE AROMATHERAPY OILS

Aromatherapy oils can be applied and enjoyed in a number of ways:

▶ *Blended with a massage oil, they can enhance massage.*

▶ *Mixed with a little water, a few drops of oil can be slowly evaporated in an incense burner to stimulate pleasant feelings.*

▶ *A few drops can be added to bath water for soothing effects.*

▶ *A soothing compress can be made by collecting a film of oil on a damp washcloth or piece of soft cotton fabric.*

▶ *Moisturizers and skin lotions can be enhanced with essential oils.*

with aromatherapy oils, which enhance the therapeutic effects of the massage.

AROMATHERAPY

There are two basic mechanisms involved in aromatherapy—the sense of smell and the absorptive quality of skin. Aromatherapy is based on the therapeutic effects of active ingredients found in the essential oils of plants, which are extracted from roots, leaves, flowers, seeds, or bark. Lavender, eucalyptus, and sage are common examples of oils recommended for the relief of physical and emotional problems.

It is known that smell is the most acute of the five senses and that certain scents can evoke memories of past events, heighten awareness, or induce changes in mood. Exactly how aromatherapy works, however, is not understood. Aromatherapists claim that the inhalation of a certain scent can prompt the brain to release neurochemicals that will counter such problems as stress and fatigue. They also believe that some oils exert a medicinal effect when absorbed by the skin.

Although many claims made for aromatherapy have yet to be substantiated in clinical trials, few who have received aromatherapy would deny that it is a highly relaxing and uplifting experience, and many would testify to its therapeutic effects on a range of conditions.

In one of its most widely practiced forms, aromatherapy consists of a whole-body massage using a base oil containing a small quantity of one or more essential oils. Hand movements are basically those of Swedish massage, with the treatment concentrated on parts of the body that store tension. Although much of the relaxing effect comes from the massage itself, this is enhanced by the essential oils. Some aromatherapists make use of this relaxed state to encourage a patient to discuss any personal problems or feelings of anxiety that may be contributing to stress or health disorders. In this way aromatherapy can comprise a deeper and more thorough treatment than it first appears.

The concept of aromatherapy is far from new. Traditional Chinese medicine has drawn on the medicinal qualities of herbs and scents for some 5,000 years. The Egyptians used herbal oils in massage and bathing, as well as for health and therapeutic purposes. Both the Greeks and Romans enjoyed the health-giving benefits of bathing in water that contained small amounts of essential oils and breathing the vapors produced by evaporating them in an oil burner.

The name *aromatherapy* comes from the French term *aromathérapie*, which was first used by René-Maurice Gattefossé, a French chemist, in a research paper published in 1928. Working in his family perfumery, Gattefossé discovered the potential healing powers of essential oils when he bathed his hand in lavender essence after burning himself badly in a laboratory accident. The therapy gained ready acceptance in France as treatment for a wide range of conditions. It was not introduced into Britain until 1969, and its rise in popularity was initially slow. Since 1985, however, it has become the most rapidly expanding form of alternative therapy in that country.

Essential oils have also become big business in North America, where they are sold in health food stores and pharmacies. For those not trained in aromatherapy who would like to treat themselves, blends of oils for specific conditions are widely available. If you plan to diagnose and treat yourself, you must exercise care, as a number of the oils are contraindicated for certain conditions (see pages 152–156). It is absolutely vital to follow the manufacturer's directions found on a bottle, particularly regarding the dilution of essential oils, which must not be exceeded under any circumstances (see Chapter 6). For anyone who wishes to know more, detailed courses are available on diagnosis and treatment.

MANUAL LYMPHATIC DRAINAGE

Manual lymphatic drainage (MLD) aims to improve the removal of impurities and bacteria from the body. It is a light stroking massage that was first devised in France in the 1930s. Under normal circumstances, the flow of lymph through the body is quite slow; it depends upon a small residual pressure from the heart and muscular contraction to push it along. MLD is designed to speed up this flow.

The predominant technique is thumb stroking, which is always directed toward the nearest lymph nodes. When treating arms or legs, a therapist starts massaging toward the lymph nodes nearest the trunk, even if the problem is near the extreme end of a limb. Treatment is unhurried and gentle and can take up to 90 minutes. The patient undresses and lies on a massage couch, with towels draped over the parts of the body that are not being treated at any given time.

MLD therapy is very relaxing and excellent for stress relief. When done regularly, it is credited with boosting the immune system and treating swelling in the tissues. However, anyone who has suffered from tuberculosis is advised against having MLD

LYMPHATIC SYSTEM

The lymphatic system consists of a network of capillaries that collect impurities from the body's tissues in lymph fluid. This travels through the system to the lymph nodes, where the impurities are filtered out for removal from the body. A massage therapist will always massage toward the nearest lymph node, thus forcing the impurities out of the tissues.

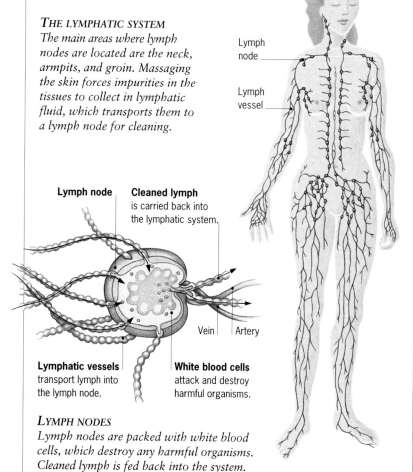

THE LYMPHATIC SYSTEM
The main areas where lymph nodes are located are the neck, armpits, and groin. Massaging the skin forces impurities in the tissues to collect in lymphatic fluid, which transports them to a lymph node for cleaning.

Lymph node

Lymph vessel

Lymph node

Cleaned lymph is carried back into the lymphatic system.

Vein | Artery

Lymphatic vessels transport lymph into the lymph node.

White blood cells attack and destroy harmful organisms.

LYMPH NODES
Lymph nodes are packed with white blood cells, which destroy any harmful organisms. Cleaned lymph is fed back into the system.

because bacterial spores lodged in the lymph nodes can be released during massage and reinfect the system.

SPORTS MASSAGE

Sports massage is a relatively recent development that combines techniques from Swedish massage, physiotherapy, chiropractic, osteopathy, kinesiology, and sometimes acupressure. It is primarily intended to maintain and enhance performance levels by detecting any muscle and tissue imbalances or weaknesses and correcting them before damage is done. Those who receive regular sports massage at the hands of an expert should be far less prone to injury.

The sports therapist uses the basic Swedish techniques of stroking, kneading, and percussion but with some important differences. Much deeper pressures are applied by using the heels of the palms, the forearms, and elbows for both stroking and kneading. The sports therapist must have a sound knowledge of anatomy and an ability to recognize and diagnose the characteristics of muscle dysfunction.

In Swedish massage, stroking is typically performed along the length of the muscles, whereas the sports therapist also massages across the muscles. Such deep stroking across muscles, known as friction, is commonly used to break down connective tissue adhesions and to help detect the exact position of fibrous and knotted tissue.

Sports masseurs also use muscle energy methods, which have their origin in applied kinesiology (see Chapter 4) and osteopathy (see Chapter 3). These are used to correct muscle imbalances and release tension by stretching muscles beyond their current capabilities. Effective treatment with muscle energy techniques involves effort and exercises on the part of the patient as well.

REMEDIAL MASSAGE

This is the use of Swedish massage methods to treat soft-tissue pain. As with sports massage, familiar techniques are used in a more penetrating way to condition deeper tissues in order to enhance recovery and return a patient to complete health.

Remedial massage can be very beneficial to those recovering from injury or surgery and can promote relaxation and all-round health. It is thought that deep massage of broken or damaged tissues improves blood

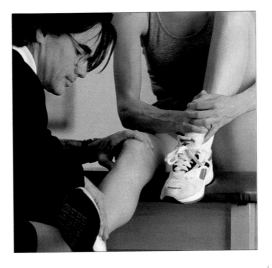

SPORTS INJURIES
A primary role of sports masseurs is to help speed recovery from sports injuries, both immediately after an injury and during long-term recovery from one.

circulation to the area, which helps to speed recovery. Another proposed explanation is that the occasional pressure on the mending tissues forces them to grow stronger and more resilient than they would have done otherwise, and at a much faster rate. It has certainly been proven that remedial massage aids recovery, but the precise reasons for this are not yet fully understood.

Remedial massage has very few contraindications, and it is used frequently in hospitals and clinics to help patients who are recovering from injuries or major surgery. It is always advisable to consult your doctor beforehand if you have any doubts about treatment or have any other conditions or illnesses that may need to be taken into consideration.

CONTRAINDICATIONS

Massage is a very safe therapy— almost entirely without negative side effects. However, there are a few medical conditions for which massage should be modified or avoided:

▶ *skin infections, inflammation, severe bruising, open wounds*

▶ *varicose veins, inflammation of the veins (phlebitis)*

▶ *deep-vein thrombosis*

▶ *cardiac disease, high blood pressure*

▶ *infectious disease, high fever*

▶ *cancer, particularly when it has invaded the lymphatic system*

▶ *undiagnosed lumps under the skin*

▶ *pregnancy*

SWEDISH MASSAGE STROKES

Swedish massage releases tensions and improves circulation, helping to speed elimination of toxins and rejuvenate body tissues. For many it also generates a good overall feeling.

The traditional techniques of Swedish massage are effleurage, petrissage, and tapotement, although they are more familiarly known as stroking, kneading, and percussion. Within each group various methods have been developed to relax muscles, relieve tension, and enhance mobility. Some of these techniques are easy to learn, so that almost anyone can give a soothing body massage at home.

STROKING
This is the traditional effleurage. The technique requires that the palm side of the hands remain in contact with the body throughout. The fingers are held together in a relaxed way as they lead the stroking hand across the skin. Even at its lightest, stroking always involves a degree of pushing. This is generated through the heels of the palms, with body weight providing the motive

STROKING *(Effleurage)*

One of the most pleasurable massage techniques, the stroke involves a long sweep of the full hands over the patient's body. It is important to keep the movements flowing.

Keep your fingers pointing forward, covering the backbone and the whole surrounding area.

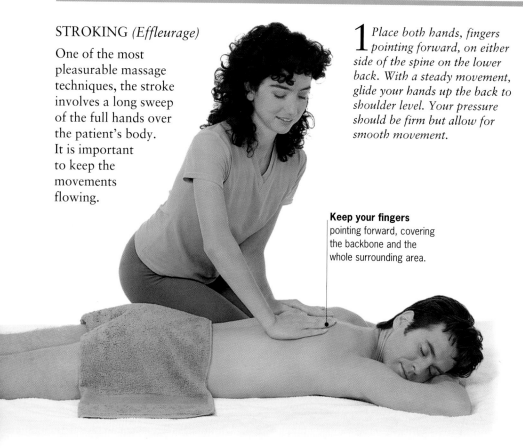

1 *Place both hands, fingers pointing forward, on either side of the spine on the lower back. With a steady movement, glide your hands up the back to shoulder level. Your pressure should be firm but allow for smooth movement.*

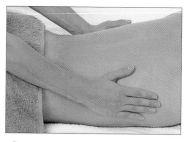

2 *Separate your hands and flow them down the sides of the body to the waist. This downward stroke should be lighter.*

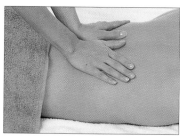

3 *Move the hands up the sides of the waist. Only when the hands draw up the lower back can pressure be slightly increased, particularly on the lowest region.*

force. At no time should any deep pressure be used with this technique.

Initial contact is made using slow, rhythmical movements, usually on the back, which is a strong area of the body, providing large surfaces of muscled tissue that benefit greatly from stroking.

Even the lightest stroking action creates friction, which produces a balmy warmth. The warmth causes dilation of blood capillaries in the skin, thus increasing blood flow. The pressure on the tissues under the skin's surface eases the connective tissue that binds the muscles.

KNEADING

Any technique that involves moving the skin against the underlying tissues is known as kneading. It is deeper and more penetrating than stroking and can be done with the palms, fingers, thumbs, or knuckles. The deepest pressure is generated when the area of application is small; for example, a thumb produces more pressure for the same force than a palm. Classical petrissage is simply kneading with the thumb. Rotations are kneading that is done with a rotating pressure. Squeezing is also a form of kneading, in which one or both hands are used to squeeze an area of skin without twisting.

Kneading is beneficial to the layers of connective tissue called fasciae, which allow muscles to move smoothly against one another as well as the surrounding tissues. When muscles become tense and knotted, the fasciae contract and start to bind tissues together. The most important effect of kneading is to release any contracted fascia so that the muscles can relax. Kneading also helps to drain lymph from the tissues near the surface and improves blood circulation.

PERCUSSION

Percussion is a series of short, sharp taps or slaps on the skin. Movements range from gentle finger tapping to a hearty pummeling, which can leave the body feeling as if it has had the daylights literally beaten out of it!

Percussion depends on vibration to release any tension from the muscles and shake

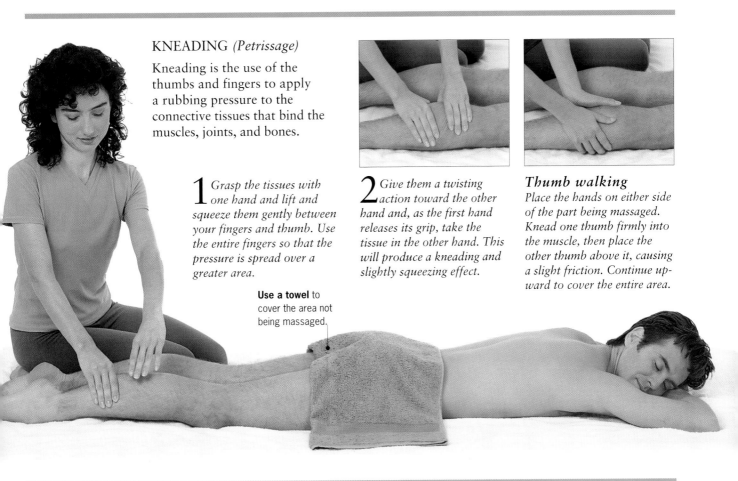

KNEADING (Petrissage)

Kneading is the use of the thumbs and fingers to apply a rubbing pressure to the connective tissues that bind the muscles, joints, and bones.

1 *Grasp the tissues with one hand and lift and squeeze them gently between your fingers and thumb. Use the entire fingers so that the pressure is spread over a greater area.*

Use a towel to cover the area not being massaged.

2 *Give them a twisting action toward the other hand and, as the first hand releases its grip, take the tissue in the other hand. This will produce a kneading and slightly squeezing effect.*

Thumb walking
Place the hands on either side of the part being massaged. Knead one thumb firmly into the muscle, then place the other thumb above it, causing a slight friction. Continue upward to cover the entire area.

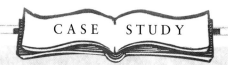
A Chronic Stress Sufferer

Stress is an all too common consequence of modern lifestyles, and many of us suffer more stress than is good for us. Stress is not just a feeling that affects us mentally and emotionally; it has an impact on almost every aspect of our physical being and, if left unchecked, can eventually cause serious medical problems.

Teresa is a 36-year-old highflier who runs her own computer software business, which has been so successful in recent years that she now has branches in different parts of the country. She travels extensively by car and spends many hours of the week in high-level meetings or working at a computer. She would describe herself as being in good health, but she does suffer from headaches, stiffness, and tense shoulder muscles.

Her relationship with her partner, James, is not going well. She knows that something needs to be done about it, but lack of time and a constant feeling of tiredness when they are together leaves the situation unresolved. This is adding to her worries considerably.

WHAT SHOULD TERESA DO?

Teresa's problems are almost all the result of her lifestyle. The tension in her neck and shoulders is most likely causing the frequent headaches. Instead of taking painkillers, she could try to control this condition by treating herself twice a week to a good massage. This is an excellent way to let go of day-to-day stresses and at the same time remove some of the knots in those muscles. At the age of 36, Teresa should not feel as stiff as she often does. Regular exercise would help limber up her body in conjunction with the massage. She must also make time to spend with her partner so that they can work through their problems and learn to enjoy their relationship more.

Action Plan

LIFESTYLE
Make provision for more time to share activities with James. Put time aside for talking and discussing the relationship.

HEALTH
Establish a regular aerobics and swimming routine. Join a health or sports club for support and encouragement.

STRESS
Have regular massage to help unwind and relieve muscle tension. Learn some relaxation techniques, such as yoga, meditation, or t'ai chi.

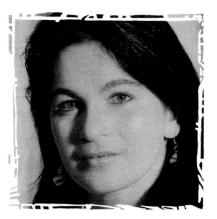

HEALTH
Frequent headaches result from neck and shoulder tension. Worry about a relationship feeds in more stress.

LIFESTYLE
A lack of time to relax properly and maintain relationships will increase stress.

STRESS
Stress on a continuous basis weakens the immune system, exposing the body to an increased likelihood of illness and further muscle tensions.

HOW THINGS TURNED OUT FOR TERESA

Teresa started to have a weekly massage, which has greatly eased the tension in her shoulders and helped her to become more relaxed. She now goes swimming twice a week and attends a weekly aerobics class, and she feels much better for the exercise. Teresa began to share her enjoyment of massage with her partner at home. This has helped to renew their intimacy and brought them closer together.

them back into their balanced and relaxed positions. Percussion strokes can be highly satisfying, although firm pummeling should not be continued for more than a few minutes without stopping briefly.

THE MASSAGE SEQUENCE

Per Henrik Ling's original system of massage is still recommended today. It should start with stroking, which allows the practitioner to spread oil evenly over the massage area and has a powerful comforting effect. As the massage partner relaxes, more pressure can gradually be applied to the stroking action. The most powerful strokes on the arms and legs should be upward ones to assist the return of blood to the heart. Traditionally, the strokes up the back are stronger than the downward ones, also encouraging blood flow back to the heart.

Kneading techniques are always used after stroking, focusing on problem areas with a deeper pressure. A return to the relaxing strokes then follows more penetrating methods. The strokes are a good way of providing a smooth link between different techniques.

More kneading could be required where tense and knotted tissues remain. Once tissues in the area being massaged are suitably relaxed, percussion strokes can be used to stimulate and tone muscles. The massage concludes with stroking, using long sweeping movements on each area of the body.

After learning the different methods, you can innovate. Try a whole-body massage using only stroking, varying the pressure and speed. You will be surprised at how enjoyable this can be. The professional, of course, will skillfully use a variety of techniques.

CARE FOR YOUR PATIENT

Swedish massage is performed on bare skin. This involves exposure of large areas of the body, and the patient's need for privacy should be respected at all times. Give the choice of wearing underpants throughout the massage. If nudity is the option chosen, keep a towel draped across the pelvic region for warmth as well as discretion. It is important to establish a trusting relationship: as you tune into each other, the communication of touch becomes more meaningful.

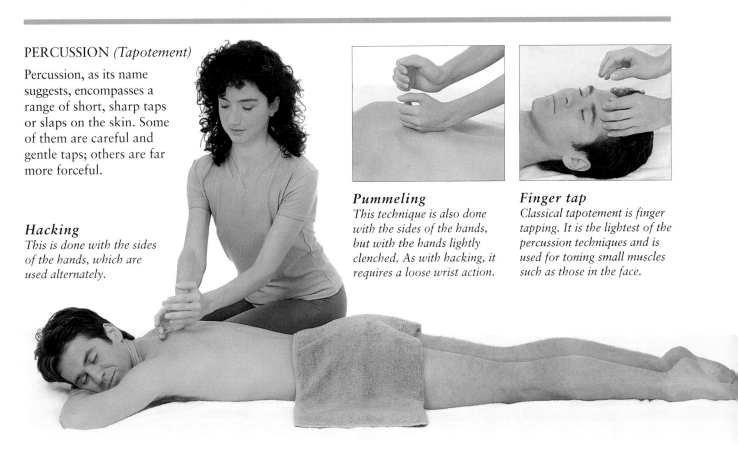

PERCUSSION *(Tapotement)*

Percussion, as its name suggests, encompasses a range of short, sharp taps or slaps on the skin. Some of them are careful and gentle taps; others are far more forceful.

Hacking
This is done with the sides of the hands, which are used alternately.

Pummeling
This technique is also done with the sides of the hands, but with the hands lightly clenched. As with hacking, it requires a loose wrist action.

Finger tap
Classical tapotement is finger tapping. It is the lightest of the percussion techniques and is used for toning small muscles such as those in the face.

Relieving muscle tension

Nobody knows the main tension areas in your body better than you, and you can use self-massage to relax them in your own home. Put 10 minutes aside a few times a week to massage tender spots and release the tension from your body.

THE HEAD AND NECK

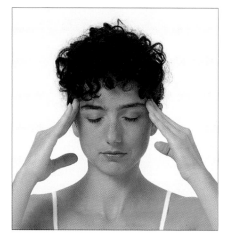 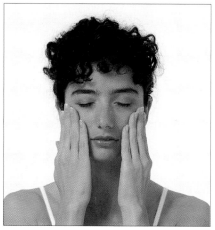 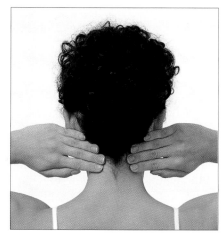

1 *From the center of your forehead, stroke outward to the hairline, then down your face to the chin.*

2 *Starting from your chin, stroke up your cheeks to the forehead. Rest your fingers on the sides of your forehead.*

3 *With your head tilted slightly forward, bring your fingers up your neck and into your hair.*

THE ARMS

1 *Use the fingers of your right hand to stroke from the back of the left hand up the arm, over the top of the shoulder, and up the side of the neck.*

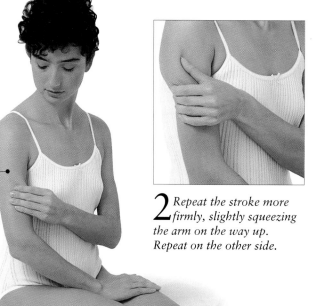

The upper arm carries a great deal of stress and should be massaged thoroughly.

2 *Repeat the stroke more firmly, slightly squeezing the arm on the way up. Repeat on the other side.*

THE HIPS

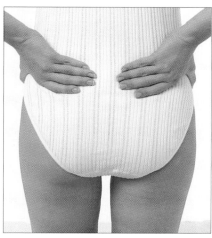

Stand up and place both hands on either side of the spine, level with the lower ribs. Stroke firmly downward onto the buttocks, and circle back over the hips to the starting point. Repeat several times. Use pressure on the downward strokes, but take care not to cause pain.

THE SHOULDER

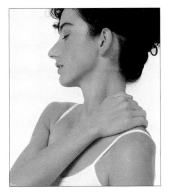

1 *Stroke firmly up your upper arm and over the shoulder. Feel where the tensions are in this area so that you can focus on them at later stages in the massage. Repeat several times.*

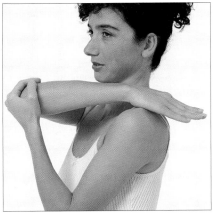

2 *Stretch your shoulder joint by taking an elbow in one hand and pulling it toward your neck. You should feel strain in the top of the arm and the joint with the shoulder. Hold for a few seconds, then repeat. Do the same with the other arm.*

3 *Knead the top of the shoulder for at least a minute to release all the tension from the muscles. This may re- quire all the strength you can muster.*

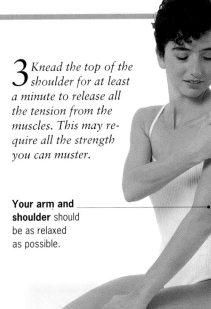

Your arm and shoulder should be as relaxed as possible.

THE LEGS

1 *Sitting up with your back straight, lean forward to grasp one leg above the ankle with both hands. Stroke up toward the top of the thigh with a pulling action on both the inner and outer sides of the leg. Repeat twice, then do the same with the other leg.*

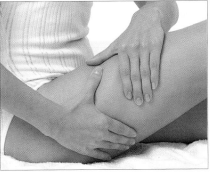

2 *With both hands, thoroughly knead all parts of the thigh that are comfortably accessible.*

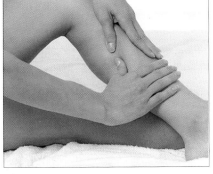

3 *Knead down your calf from your knee, paying particular attention to the calf muscles running down the leg.*

KNEADING THE FOOT

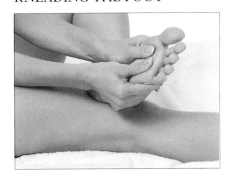

Fully massage the foot, kneading thoroughly from the heel up to the toes. Roll the toes between your fingers.

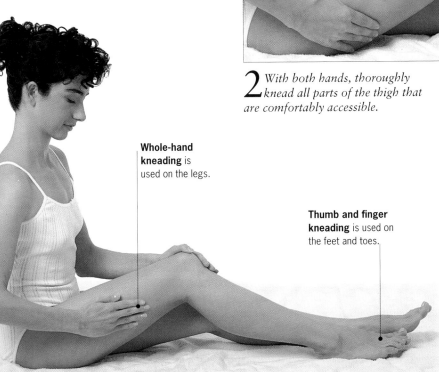

Whole-hand kneading is used on the legs.

Thumb and finger kneading is used on the feet and toes.

TYPES OF EASTERN MASSAGE

Eastern massage systems are now becoming popular all over the world. At their root is the belief that true health is based on the harmonious interaction of body and mind.

An ancient tradition in the East, massage has been enjoyed for millennia, as much for the sensual pleasure of it as for the numerous health and beauty benefits. There are hundreds of massage variations, with a range of different techniques and systems, each derived from its own culture. The styles outlined on the following pages will vary in practice from one region to another and according to a practitioner's skills and background.

INDIAN MASSAGE

There are more varieties of massage to be found on the Indian subcontinent than anywhere else in the world. Some serve

THE AYURVEDIC SYSTEM

Massage forms part of the traditional Indian system of medicine called Ayurveda, which also includes exercise, diet adjustments, and physical treatments. According to this system, each person is made up of a combination of three life energies, or doshas—called Kapha, Pitta, and Vata—with one form dominating. This dominant dosha determines personality type and also influences one's susceptibility to certain illnesses. Your frame, pulse rate, personality, and dominant body organ all reveal your principal dosha.

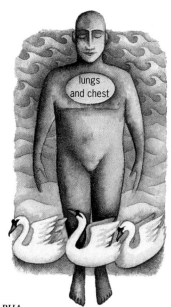

KAPHA
Characteristics: thick-framed, calm, lethargic, loving, greedy, possessive, envious. Pulse moves like a swan (50–70 beats per minute).

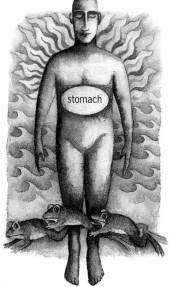

PITTA
Characteristics: medium-framed, confident, hateful, aggressive, sharp, intelligent, jealous. Pulse jumps like a frog (70–90 beats per minute).

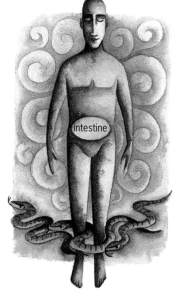

VATA
Characteristics: small-framed, emotional, restless, creative, nervous, anxious, alert, insecure. Pulse moves like a snake (90–110 beats per minute).

therapeutic purposes, while others are for pleasure primarily. There are endless varieties of body work, ranging from soft-tissue massage to manipulative therapies. It is even possible to find a whole-body massage performed only with the feet.

Most Indian massage practices today have roots in the ancient Ayurvedic system of health care, which depends on massage therapies to promote general health and longevity and to balance three basic life energies, or doshas (see opposite page).

It is recommended that massage be taken regularly and with certain oils to treat dosha imbalances. For example, if you have a Vata condition, massage should be performed in the evening with sesame oil blends, stroking against the grain of the skin for extra penetration. For a Pitta disorder, take massage in the afternoon using sunflower or sandalwood oil for their cooling properties. If you are suffering from a kapha disorder, you should have a massage in the morning with corn oil or no oil at all.

Indian head massage
Many tourists have returned from India enthused about the wonders of a head massage tried there. This is available in Western countries but not widely; if you are seeking it, make sure that the masseur is properly trained or well-experienced.

Traditionally, the head massage is performed with aromatic oils on the neck, scalp, and face. Many practitioners in the West extend the area of application to include the shoulders, which can store large amounts of tension. There is no need to undress, and the massage is done with the patient comfortably seated in a chair. Squeezing, rubbing, kneading, and stroking techniques are all used, together with some firm tugging of handfuls of hair.

Almost everybody can enjoy and benefit from Indian head massage. Only those with

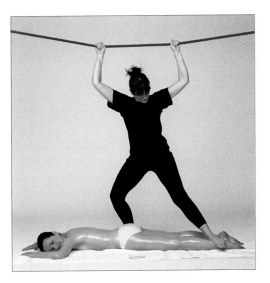

INDIAN MASSAGE
In Chavutti Thirumal massage, the practitioner treads all over the patient's body, supported from above by a rope or bar. Practitioners are highly trained, because the techniques used can be dangerous if they are not fully understood or correctly applied.

skin conditions affecting the scalp, such as psoriasis and eczema, should avoid it.

Most people say they feel wonderful after an Indian head massage. It is very good for treating headaches, sinus problems, and neck pains. Regular head massage is reputed to encourage strong, lustrous hair growth and facial skin that glows with good health.

Chavutti Thirumal massage
This southern Indian technique could hardly be more different from head massage. It is performed with the feet only on the oiled body of the subject, who lies naked on a towel on the floor, although underwear is sometimes worn. A bar or rope is suspended overhead, and the masseur holds onto it to control the amount of weight applied. There is nothing rough or uncontrolled about the massage: it takes years of training and practical experience to master.

With wonderfully coordinated movements, the therapist strokes, kneads, and squeezes the patient's body, massaging all parts, including the hands, feet, and face. Since considerable pressure is often applied, there may be some brief discomfort. This is most often felt when the backs of the legs and buttocks are treated. A full-body massage can take up to one and a half hours. It is better not to make any plans for activities immediately afterward, as you may feel drowsy or tired while your body readjusts to the release of strains and tensions.

Chavutti is an excellent therapy for serious stress relief. Back and shoulder pain, sciatica, and headaches of all kinds respond well. Unfortunately, few practitioners work outside the Indian subcontinent.

CAUTION
Chavutti Thirumal is not for the weak-hearted. Do not consider taking this massage unless your body is in good physical condition and you are strong enough to cope with a thorough pummeling.

The Thai Masseur

Thai massage is a healing system that aims to maintain the body's physical condition and to calm and balance the emotions. Even the most stressed individual can emerge from a Thai massage with a feeling of lightness and relaxation.

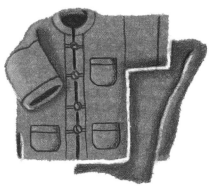

THAI CLOTHING
Many Thai masseurs wear traditional clothing consisting of a dark blue cotton top and loose trousers.

Origins

Thai massage stems directly from Buddhism and is believed to have been developed in northern India by Jivaka Bhaccha, physician to the Buddha, around 600 BC. It was used only by monks until the 19th century, when King Rama III of Thailand ordered the techniques to be brought to the temple of Wat Pho in Bangkok. From there the massage spread throughout Thailand.

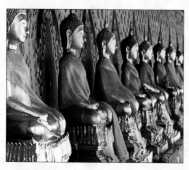

WAT PHO
The massage techniques were described in stone carvings, which can be seen in the important Buddhist temple of Wat Pho.

How does Thai massage differ from Western massage?

Thai massage involves the most complex physical interaction between giver and receiver of any massage available. Even though the participants are fully clothed throughout, traditional Thai massage is the ultimate nonsexual touch experience. Only a few techniques are used, and most of the sequence is based on stretches and manipulations incorporating pressure. Through precise position, balance, and use of body weight, the masseur achieves what looks like effortless leverage. Quite often the receiver of the massage must cooperate and work with the masseur to create the desired effects.

The soft-tissue treatments used in Western massage, including the uses of oil or talcum powder on the bare skin, seem static by comparison. Even sports massage depends on few manipulation techniques. Thai massage contributes to high levels of flexibility, while Western massage has little to offer in this respect.

What happens during a session of Thai massage?

The room will have a massage mat set out on the floor. You will be asked some questions about the condition of your health to make sure you have no health problems that could contraindicate the treatment. The Thai masseur should be able to work the massage around most problems

THAI MASSAGE
The practitioner uses stretches and pulls to create a balance likened to a harmonious duet between the patient and the masseur.

if you explain the nature of the condition in full.

The massage will begin with you lying on your back in a relaxed position. The sequence starts at your feet: this part of the treatment is very thorough and feels much like reflexology, but it is only the beginning. Each leg is then massaged in turn, with lots of palming and deep thumb walking along the energy lines. Both legs are manipulated, helping to relax the hips and lower back. Next, the abdomen, chest, and arms are treated. The pace is unhurried; Thai masseurs act as if time is of no importance.

At this point, you will be asked to turn onto your side, and each side will be treated in turn. Every part that is accessible in this position will now receive detailed attention. With the changed position, you may hardly recognize that some of the techniques are repetitions of ones used earlier. When the treatment has been completed on both sides, you will change position again and lie face down. Everything that is exposed—feet, legs, buttocks, back, arms, and hands—will be pressed, kneaded, stretched, and manipulated.

You will probably feel reluctant to assume the sitting position required for the final section of the massage, which treats the neck, shoulders, head, and face.

The unique feature of Thai massage is that every part of the body is massaged and manipulated in a variety of positions. To experience the greatest benefits of this type of massage you must be able to relax completely in order to let the tensions and stresses be released from your body.

What should I wear?

You should wear lightweight cotton clothing that covers your legs and arms and remove your shoes and socks. The masseur will also be wearing lightweight cotton clothes and will be barefoot. Do not wear jewelry, and keep your hair tied back if it is long.

What conditions does it treat?

Headaches and pain or tension in the neck, shoulders, back, and hips all respond to the Thai therapist's touch. Many who receive regular massage report improved sleep, and sciatica sufferers enjoy relief from their pains. Joint mobility and muscle tone are increased, and thus posture is improved. On the emotional level, the massage has a general calming effect.

What training should a Thai masseur have?

A professional Thai masseur should have a diploma from a recognized massage therapy institute (most have learned Swedish massage). In addition, he or she will have studied basic Thai massage techniques for at least 200 hours, and perhaps will have additional training in advanced methods. There are Thai masseurs who have learned their skills from masters in Thailand, many of whom have no formal qualifications, so word of mouth is often the best means of finding a good masseur.

Who can benefit from a Thai massage?

Almost anyone can benefit from a traditional Thai massage. The main exceptions are women in the later stages of pregnancy and the very frail, particularly people suffering from osteoporosis. A skilled therapist should be able to adapt the massage to accommodate most types of physical disability or other illnesses and conditions.

AFTER TOUCH THERAPY

A good time to meditate is when the body and mind are relaxed after a massage. The general aim is to clear the mind by concentrating on one thing to the exclusion of all else. One simple method is to focus on the inhaling and exhaling of your breath. This becomes easier the more you practice, so don't give up if it doesn't come to you right away.

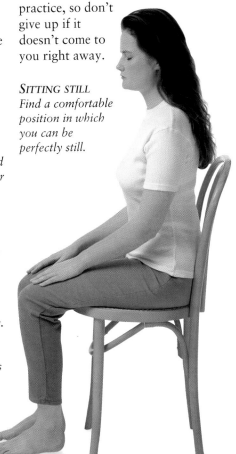

SITTING STILL
Find a comfortable position in which you can be perfectly still.

1 *Make sure that you are in a comfortable position, ideally sitting up straight. Relax your body, feeling the release of tensions.*

2 *Begin to focus on your breathing and count your breaths as they leave your body. Count to 10 and then start again at 1. Continue this for about 5 minutes.*

3 *Start to count your breaths as they enter your body, again from 1 to 10. Continue this for about 5 minutes.*

4 *Concentrate on realizing the first point at which you feel the breath and the last at which it leaves your body. Feel it filling your chest and expanding and contracting your ribs. Consider the texture of the air and any other sensations as you become aware of them.*

5 *When you have finished, slowly allow your normal thoughts to return, remaining still and relaxed and retaining a sense of calm.*

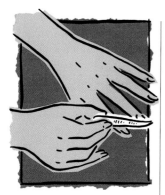

IMPROVING YOUR TOUCH

Manicuring your hands regularly can help you improve your sense of touch. Massage the joints and muscles and around the cuticles, feeling their shapes and the condition of the skin. File the fingernails carefully and then treat your skin to a good moisturizer.

The very frail and those suffering from heart problems, seriously high blood pressure, epilepsy, and cancer should avoid this type of massage.

THAI TRADITIONAL MASSAGE

The recent growth in tourism to Thailand has led to a surge of interest in traditional Thai massage, which draws on the spiritual balance and ancient practices of Buddhist philosophy. It is performed on the floor, with the client fully clothed, and is rather like applied yoga, aiming for mental and emotional relaxation while pursuing whole-body flexibility.

Thai massage has Buddhist origins but draws on a number of other sources for its methodology, including elements of the Indian Ayurvedic and Yogic systems, as well as Chinese Tuina. It has probably existed in roughly its present form for over a thousand years. It is based on the body's energy channels, called sen, but with far less precision than in the practice of traditional Chinese medicine. Hands, elbows, knees, and feet are used to massage and manipulate the body into an extraordinary number of different positions.

It is suitable for most people, with the exception of those who have any of the conditions listed on page 43. Additionally,

conditions listed on page 43.

DID YOU KNOW?
Pacific island massages were enjoyed by Captain James Cook and his crew in the late 18th century. This method of health care, in addition to nutritional considerations, enabled Cook to keep most of his crew alive and healthy throughout his expeditions.

it is not appropriate for anyone who has artificial hip or knee joints or who has undergone surgery during the past six months. All manipulations involving the back should be avoided by those who have had major surgery on the spine or who suffer from severe back problems.

Thai massage can be of huge benefit both physically and emotionally. By having joints moved through a range of movements that are all just a little more than the receiver would be capable of unaided, the body becomes more supple. Intrinsic body energies are balanced to promote pain-free, good health. The greatest benefits from this unique type of massage come to those who are able to relax totally and can be fully manipulated by the masseur.

INDONESIAN MASSAGE

Dating back at least 2,000 years, Indonesian massage has elements that are akin to some in Ayurveda and the main energy meridians of traditional Chinese medicine. Whether this is the result of Chinese and Indian influence in the distant past, or whether Indonesia developed its system independently, it is difficult to say. The massage is deep and is definitely not for the faint-hearted. For those seeking the ultimate penetrating oil massage, however, this could well be it.

Treatment is performed on the floor or on a hard bed or couch. The recipient is naked but may be partially covered with a towel over areas that are not receiving attention. Indonesian masseurs have astonishing strength in their thumbs, their principal massage tool. Even the stroking techniques are penetrating, made as they are with the heels of the palms and lots of body weight to push deeply into the tissues. Thumb kneading is used over the entire body to release deep-muscle tension. Stretches, pulls, and twists produce a stress-relieving effect in the spine and shoulders, leaving the recipient feeling unburdened and invigorated.

BUDDHISM

The strong Buddhist influence in Thai traditional massage represents "the giving of loving care." Nonaggression and compassion for all living things are among the principal tenets of Buddhist philosophy. Traditionally practiced in temples by Buddhist monks, this massage method was used to enhance spiritual detachment from the world and all its material desires, thus helping the monks to achieve enlightenment. In this sense, Thai massage can be seen as a spiritually uplifting treatment that enables a person to achieve a sense of objectivity and higher reasoning.

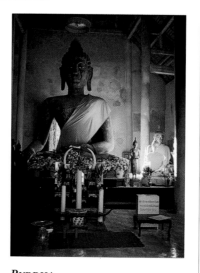

BUDDHA
The image of Buddha embodies the meditative calmness that is reflected in Buddhist Thai massage.

Not surprisingly, this massage is not recommended for those with the usual conditions that would contraindicate any kind of massage (see page 43). Its appeal could well be further limited, however, because of its intensity and depth, which can be quite painful at times.

Indonesian massage offers a range of techniques for treating chronic and acute muscle and joint pain. It can calm the emotions, relax the body and mind, and contribute to an overall feeling of well being. Headaches, sciatica, and insomnia respond well.

As practiced today, Indonesian massage is still very much part of an effective healing system that also includes herbal remedies, known as Jamu. Herbs and spices have always played a large and important role in Eastern health and therapeutic remedies. Jamu includes traditional healing with stimulating and soothing ingredients such as ginger, lemongrass, and coconut milk.

HAWAIIAN MASSAGE (LOMI LOMI)

This traditional massage comes from the islands of Polynesia and dates back thousands of years. The massage itself is an expression of a complex Polynesian philosophy. Although it is powerfully relaxing, this is not its intended purpose: it has great religious and healing significance and for much of its history has been performed only within the family. In 1973 Aunty Margaret Machado began teaching the techniques publicly, and hundreds of her students now teach and practice the art in other countries.

The philosophy behind Hawaiian massage is so complex, few Westerners really understand its aims completely. What is clear is that it makes recipients feel relaxed and at one with the world and with their own body and inner self.

Aromatic oils are employed, and the massage is done on a massage table using palms, thumbs, and forearms in a rhythmic fashion that resembles a dance. The aim is to stimulate circulation and break up muscle spasms. In fact, Lomi Lomi means "to break up into small pieces." A whole-body massage session can take up to two hours.

Hawaiian massage is not suitable for those who suffer from any of the conditions listed on page 43 but is otherwise a quite safe and enjoyable experience. It can be used to treat tension and chronic pain in the soft tissues and the usual tender spots—such

ROSE BODY LOTION

If you apply this lotion just before going to bed, you will give the moisturizing elements time to sink deep into your skin overnight, leaving it supple and nourished for the new day.

15 g (½ oz) anhydrous lanolin
15 g (½ oz) cocoa butter
20 ml (4 tsp) almond oil

20 ml (4 tsp) glycerine
  (preferably vegetable)
6 drops rose essential oil

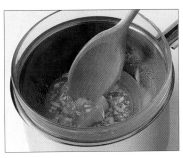
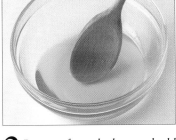

1 *Place a heatproof bowl in a saucepan of simmering water. Melt the lanolin and cocoa butter in the bowl and mix them to a smooth paste.*

2 *Remove from the heat and add the almond oil and glycerine. Stir thoroughly, allow to cool, and then add the rose essential oil, blending it in well.*

3 *Store the mixture in a small jar or bottle and use it during massage. It is also beneficial for dry or problem skin when applied before bedtime to allow complete absorption and moisturization during the night.*

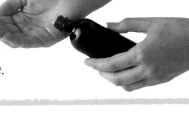

as the neck, the shoulders, and the lower back—all of which respond well.

Hawaiian massage is traditionally taught one-on-one; to master the method, a student should have at least 500 hours of instruction and apprenticeship. In the United States, only about 10 states license the practice. Most therapists must meet local requirements. There are a small number of Hawaiian massage practitioners in Canada who have learned their skills either on the U.S. mainland or in Hawaii itself. The best way to locate a person who specializes in Lomi Lomi is to find a massage therapy institute that teaches it and ask for a recommendation.

Yoga

Back pain is often caused by stresses and strains, the results of poor posture, twisting when picking something up, or bending over awkwardly. It can be avoided by regularly doing exercises that stretch and strengthen the abdominal and back muscles.

CONTRAINDICATIONS

Don't try these stretches if you have had persistent or serious back trouble. Do each exercise until you feel the strain; do not push yourself and do not stretch if you feel any pain. If you have a back problem and would like to exercise, it is best to ask your doctor or therapist for advice first.

Put aside 5 minutes every day or a few times a week for these simple stretches. They can relieve pain and keep your back flexible and supple, helping to prevent future back problems. All you need is a little space where you will not be disturbed for a few moments. Before or after a warm bath is a good time to stretch all the tensions out of your lower back. Although you need to hold the stretches for at least several seconds to obtain the best results, stop immediately if you feel pain.

THE HERO, COBRA, AND CORPSE POSES

THE HERO
Kneel with feet and knees together and a rolled towel placed at the join between your body and legs. Bend over until you can rest your arms and forehead on the floor. Hold for at least 1 minute.

Head should lean downward, with your forehead resting on the floor.

Hands should be relaxed and flat on the floor.

Elbows should be bent.

THE COBRA
Lie on your abdomen, with the palms of your hands flat on the floor just beneath your shoulders and fingers pointing toward your chin.

Raise your head, arch your neck backward, and lift your shoulders off the floor. Hold for a few seconds, then release. Rest for a minute between stretches.

Head should be held up, facing the ceiling.

Calves should be at right angles to the thighs and thighs at right angles to the body.

Arms should be relaxed at the sides of the body.

THE CORPSE POSE
In this version of the corpse pose, a chair is used to stretch the lower back. Lie down with your buttocks at the base of a chair and place your lower legs and feet on the seat. Adjust your position so you are resting comfortably with thighs at right angles to your body and lower legs at right angles to your thighs. Hold for a few minutes, breathing deeply.

EASTERN MASSAGE TECHNIQUES

Eastern massage methods, exemplified by the flowing Thai strokes described below, differ from Western approaches by their emphasis on spiritual and emotional balance and rhythm.

Nowhere is the difference between Eastern and Western massage more dramatically illustrated than in Thai massage, which feels and looks more like applied yoga than our traditional concept of massage. Many of the movements involve close, sometimes intimate, contact between the giver and receiver, and although relaxed, the receiver must often cooperate with the masseur to achieve the desired result. Wonderful shapes unfold, to be held for a few seconds before they evaporate away or blend into the next sequence. The impression given to an observer of a Thai massage could be described as a beautifully choreographed sequence of movements.

STRETCHING THE FEET

Giving the feet a good stretch can help induce relaxation, increase the flow of blood around the feet, and stimulate the muscles and skin. It can also improve mobility and flexibility, thus releasing blockages caused by tension.

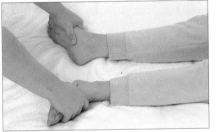

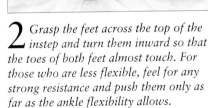

1 *The recipient's heels should be placed slightly apart. Press with your palms on the inner side of both heels. Use a gentle rocking motion and move your hands outward toward the toes.*

2 *Grasp the feet across the top of the instep and turn them inward so that the toes of both feet almost touch. For those who are less flexible, feel for any strong resistance and push them only as far as the ankle flexibility allows.*

3 *Place your palms on top of the toes and press them firmly downward so that the feet become strongly arched. Press carefully if the recipient is very stiff or in any pain.*

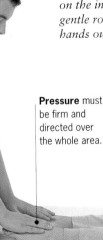

Pressure must be firm and directed over the whole area.

The body should be relaxed and the limbs flexible to the stretches.

Within a full massage, there seem to be endless nuances of tempo and pressure and a large number and variety of stretches and positions to be drawn from.

STRETCHES

Stretching out muscles and joints is central to Thai massage. This works on the principle that energy becomes trapped in these areas and needs to be dislodged through flexing and stretching. Putting slight pressure on the joints and muscles can improve all-round flexibility, allowing better ease of movement and enabling the joint to become stronger and more tolerant to everyday stresses and strains.

Manipulations are done by putting pressure on one part of the body, using one or both hands, a thumb, an elbow, knee, or the feet, and having the floor as a basis for resistance. The gentle pressures (and resulting pulling) cause the muscles to stretch and the joints to loosen and relax.

All the positions must be maneuvered slowly, without any sudden jerks or fast stretches, which may result in strains. Don't overstretch the recipient; he or she must tell you to stop straight away

CAUTION
Unless the giver weighs much less than the receiver, full body weight should not be used in Thai massage. Also, a masseur never stands directly on the spine. Standing on any part of the body requires extensive training and should never be practiced without proper guidance.

if there is any amount of pain. Generally, the stretches should be held for about 20 seconds and then released gradually over another 10 seconds.

Balancing forces

The art of stretching involves a delicate balance between the forces of the push, or the masseur's pressure, and the pulling forces, or the pull from inside the patient's body. When a balance is found, then the stretch is complete. An experienced Thai masseur understands the nuances of the push-and-pull balance and is able to apply exactly the right pressure by gauging the response.

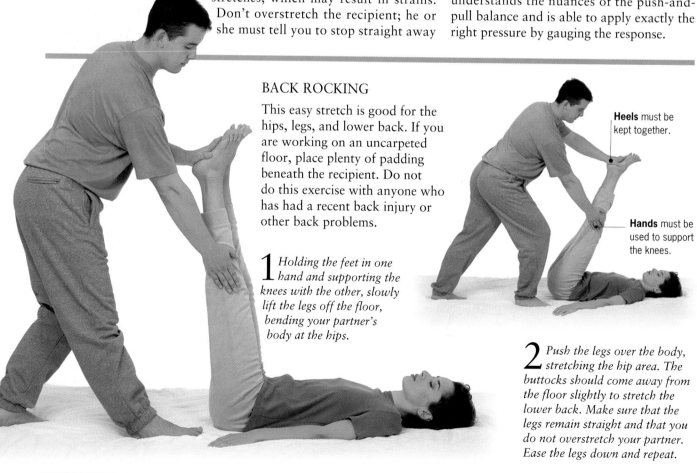

BACK ROCKING

This easy stretch is good for the hips, legs, and lower back. If you are working on an uncarpeted floor, place plenty of padding beneath the recipient. Do not do this exercise with anyone who has had a recent back injury or other back problems.

1 *Holding the feet in one hand and supporting the knees with the other, slowly lift the legs off the floor, bending your partner's body at the hips.*

Heels must be kept together.

Hands must be used to support the knees.

2 *Push the legs over the body, stretching the hip area. The buttocks should come away from the floor slightly to stretch the lower back. Make sure that the legs remain straight and that you do not overstretch your partner. Ease the legs down and repeat.*

SOFT-TISSUE TECHNIQUES

The pressure that tissues receive depends on what part of the body is used to apply it. Force applied with the thumb or tip of the elbow is much more intense than pressure created by using the whole hand or foot.

Thumb pressure

Pressure is applied with the pad of the thumb, never with the tip. This technique is potentially capable of the most concentrated pressure. It is used over areas where tension can build up between small joints or ligaments, such as the joints of the backbone, or within larger muscles. For example, it is effective for a deeper massage of the muscles running down the back of the calf on the lower leg.

Thumb walking is a method used often in Thai massage. With the thumbs in line with each other and a distance of about 3 centimeters (1 inch) between their tips, the right thumb is brought to the left one, which is now moved back 3 centimeters and applied with pressure to the body. This technique is most often used on the backbone, although it is useful for deep soft-tissue massage on other parts of the body.

Hand pressure

The simplest way to press is with the hand placed palm downward with fingers together. Pressure is generated through the therapist's body weight, which is brought over the hand after it has been placed. This should be done gently at first, with pressure being increased gradually until maximum effect is achieved. The pressure should be released progressively, and at no time should the smooth action of the therapist's body be disturbed. To achieve greater pressure, both hands are used, one on top of the other.

Elbow pressure

The elbow is used to press into areas of thick muscle, such as the tops of the shoulders and the buttocks. In some cases a little less pressure is required than that from the elbow tip. In this instance the surface of the upper forearm is used. Care must be taken when using the elbows, as they can cause a great deal of pain if applied carelessly.

Foot pressure

Feet often replace hands in Thai massage. In some cases the pressure is generated from the legs; in others the body part is pulled

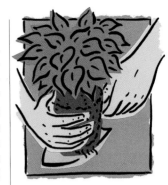

IMPROVING YOUR TOUCH

Farmers and pedologists (people who study soil) depend largely on touch to assess the condition of their soils. When you are gardening or potting household plants, rub the soil or compost through your fingers to get used to it. With experience, you will be able to gauge by touch how good the soil is for growing plants.

LEG STRETCH

Stretching the legs and feet helps to realign the joints and relieve muscle tension. Avoid this stretch if you have any ankle, knee, or leg complaints or injuries, and make sure that you do not overstretch.

1 *Kneeling on the right side of your partner, put her foot over her left leg and place your right foot over hers to keep it in place. Take the right knee in your right hand.*

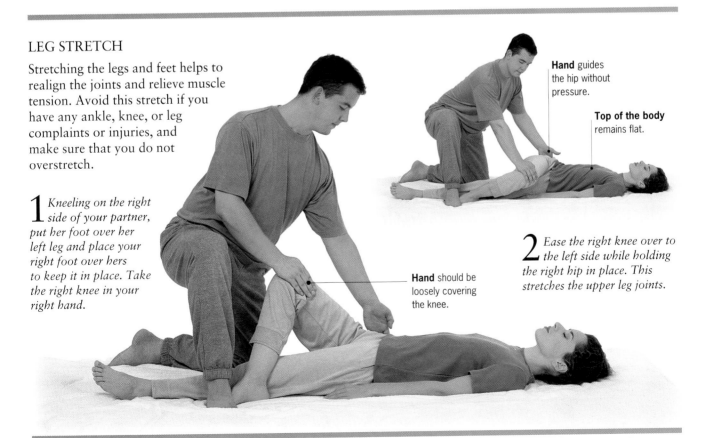

Hand guides the hip without pressure.

Top of the body remains flat.

Hand should be loosely covering the knee.

2 *Ease the right knee over to the left side while holding the right hip in place. This stretches the upper leg joints.*

against the sole of the foot. This second technique requires very careful control over the pressure that is used. The most extreme pressure from the feet comes from standing directly on the subject, which the nonprofessional should avoid. A therapist uses some kind of support to maintain control over the amount of body weight applied.

Sitting pressure

Part or all of the upper body weight can be brought to bear on the receiver by controlled sitting, in which more or less of the weight is taken on the therapist's feet or knees. Sitting is used on the buttocks and feet. Special care must be taken when performing any of these movements.

Benefits of pressure

Pressure can be applied to large areas to stimulate the sense organs and give the recipient pleasant, comforting feelings. Too much pressure can cause discomfort or pain. The well-trained therapist will know exactly the right balance of pressure to use. When sustained, pressure affects the underlying tissues so that the flow of energy is boosted. It also encourages the drainage of lymph by squeezing lymph out of the area being pressed and allowing it to flush back when pressure is released. A similar effect is achieved with blood in the surface vessels. Pressure that is deep and concentrated on a small area is ideal for breaking down knotted tissue associated with tense muscles.

SAFETY FOR THE THERAPIST

In many Thai movements the body weight of the masseur is used to counterbalance the weight of that part of the subject's body being lifted. Every movement requires balance, proper posture, and control on the part of the masseur in order to avoid straining or possibly incurring injury. Never attempt extensive lifts on anyone who is a great deal heavier or larger than you.

PRESSURE TECHNIQUES

The pressure that tissues receive depends on which part of the body is used to apply it. A force applied through the tip of the elbow or pad of the thumb will be more intense than the same force applied through the palm or sole of the foot. Although firm-pressured massage can be very relaxing, it can also be painful; the recipient must tell you if she is in any pain.

Elbow

The elbow is used to press into areas of thick muscle, such as the tops of the shoulders and the buttocks. Use gentle pressure at first to ensure that you are not causing discomfort, and then lean over your elbow to apply more weight.

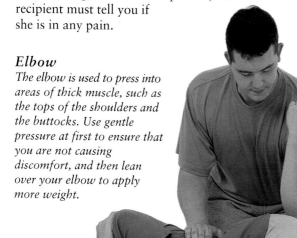

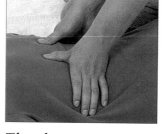

Thumb
Pressure is applied with the pad of the thumb, never with the tip, and can create an intense localized pressure.

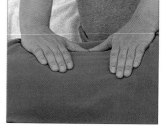

Hand
Pressure comes from the therapist's body weight, which is brought over the hand after it has been placed.

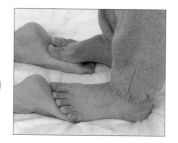

Foot
Foot pressure is generated from the masseur's legs, or the receiver's body part is pulled against the soles of the therapist's feet. The therapist can be sitting down against a wall to control the pressure.

CHAPTER 3

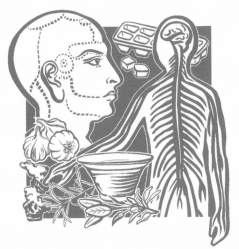

MANIPULATIVE THERAPIES

Encompassing a wide range of manipulation, stretching, and exercise techniques, manipulative therapies aim to realign the physical structure of the body to restore health and balance. A properly functioning body will help you stay relaxed and energetic, supplying you with the basic requirements for a healthy life.

OSTEOPATHY

Osteopaths work with the skeleton to alleviate muscle and joint pain. They also aim to improve the function of the skeletal frame, which relaxes tensions and promotes general good health.

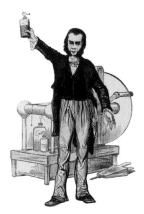

ALTERNATIVE REVIVAL
The 1870s were a heyday for natural therapies, reviving traditional liniments, ointments, and bonesetting practices for the treatment of a range of ailments.

Among alternative therapies involving physical manipulation, osteopathy has become one of the most widely used in the Western world. It is particularly popular for treating back problems and joint disorders. Since 1972, when they were recognized as fully qualified physicians, the number of doctors of osteopathy in the United States has more than doubled.

ORIGINS
Osteopathy was founded by Andrew Taylor Still, a doctor working on the Missouri frontier in the late 19th century. He believed that all the body's systems, including the musculoskeletal system, work together and that disturbances in one system may impact functions elsewhere. Still also recognized the body's self-healing capacity and believed that when disease occurred, applying corrective manipulations could help the body restore itself to good health.

TRAINING
A doctor of osteopathic medicine (D.O.) completes four years of medical training, with special emphasis on the musculoskeletal system and manipulative therapies. Like other physicians, D.O.s also do a one-year internship and a hospital residency in any of more than 120 specialties, but more than 60 percent remain in primary-care practice

Only a few osteopaths practice in Canada. Those who do, have usually trained at recognized colleges of osteopathic medicine in the United States and so are fully licensed doctors. (Canadians who have diplomas in manual osteopathy from a university may not be licensed physicians.)

PHILOSOPHY AND METHOD
The body depends on the skeletal system in order to move, walk, sit, or stand. The burden of carrying the body is put on the joints and muscles, and misalignments or other problems can occur easily. One goal of osteopathy is to restore correct positioning of the bones and relieve tensions in the joints.

First of all, the osteopath will listen carefully to a description of your problem and how it occurred. A full structural survey will then follow, during which the D.O. will ask you to adopt various positions or perform certain movements in order to assess your posture. By watching carefully, he can detect misalignments of joints, poor posture, and weak muscle areas that may be forcing other, stronger areas to compensate.

TECHNIQUES
The general methods used in osteopathy fall into four categories: soft-tissue techniques, articulatory techniques, functional treat-

---

BONESETTING

Bonesetting, the treatment of broken bones and dislocated limbs by manipulation, is a forerunner of osteopathy. Practiced for hundreds of years, it reached a peak in the 18th and 19th centuries. Bonesetting was particularly popular in rural areas, where practitioners were often an inexpensive, informal, and accessible alternative to a doctor. Treatment involved a range of manipulations, massage, and pressure techniques based both on traditional knowledge and on the intuition of the practitioner. The skill was usually passed down within a family, and most bonesetters had another occupation, often as a blacksmith or a farmer. No formal study was involved; a watch-and-practice method was used instead.

ment, and visceral techniques. Soft-tissue techniques involve manipulation of muscles. An osteopath does not use oil, as it can cause the hands to slip, and it is important to grasp the whole width of a muscle. These methods relax muscles and improve circulation.

Articulatory techniques, such as high-velocity thrusts, are manipulations used to ease movement in stiff joints. These usually include quick maneuvers, which often produce an audible crack from the joint being treated. Osteopaths call this a correction because they are correcting a problem and returning the person to health.

Functional treatment is aimed at restoring normal structure and function to fasciae, the layers of tissue that surround and connect the muscles, bones, skin, and organs. The treatment may start anywhere in the body, and the osteopath follows a fascia as it unwinds and relaxes.

Visceral technique is similar to functional treatment, but the osteopath directs the efforts at the internal organs, collectively known as the viscera. The technique usually focuses on the abdomen, mainly dealing with menstrual pain and disorders of the kidneys and bladder.

Cranial osteopathy is carried out by osteopaths who specialize in the cranial field. It is based on the concept that there are rhythms within the cranium that regulate the body. By subtly massaging the cranial bones and influencing the way they move, the osteopath adjusts and controls these rhythms in order to restore health.

PROBLEMS TREATED

Although osteopaths treat the entire spectrum of human disease, osteopathy is most commonly used for back and neck problems in which the spine seems to have clicked out of place. Arthritis and other joint problems can also be treated effectively, as can irritable bowel syndrome and other tensions in the abdomen, such as menstrual problems. Migraine and other headaches are helped particularly with cranial osteopathy.

CONTRAINDICATIONS

Before beginning manipulations, an osteopath will ask you in detail about your condition and any other problems you may have. The treatment that follows will be worked around what you have discussed, so in effect, osteopathy has no contraindications.

BODY STRETCHES

Because it improves muscle tone and flexibility, stretching is one of the best ways to keep the body healthy. When you stretch muscles and ligaments, you stimulate circulation and relieve muscle tension. These stretches are particularly good for the neck, back, and shoulders. They should be done smoothly, taking care not to jerk or overstretch.

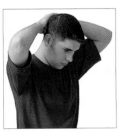

NECK AND SHOULDER STRETCH Put your chin down to your chest. Loosely clasp your hands behind your head and gently pull your head down. Feel the stretch in the muscles on the back of your neck and upper back.

UPPER BACK AND CHEST STRETCH Put your hands together in a praying position. Press them together, pushing your elbows away from your body and your shoulders forward. Feel the stretch across your shoulders and chest.

SHOULDER STRETCH Stand with your legs apart and your hands clasped behind your back. Bend over at the hips, bringing your hands up behind, which will cause you to bend farther. Feel the stretch in your shoulders and spine.

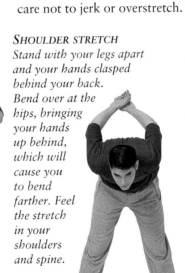

SPINE STRETCH Take a deep breath and raise your arms above your head. Slowly lean back so that you are looking at your hands; you will feel your spine and neck being stretched.

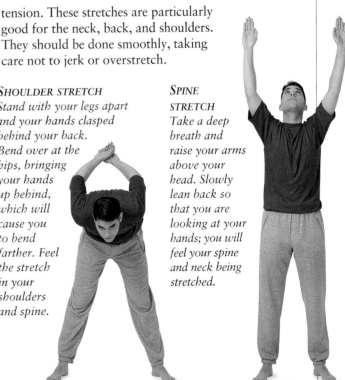

The Osteopath

A misalignment of the spine can affect your whole body, throwing your sense of balance into disarray and disturbing your overall well-being. Osteopathy aims to restore musculoskeletal flexibility and return you to complete health.

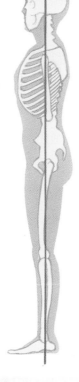

PERFECT POSTURE
Part of osteopathic diagnosis and treatment involves an analysis of posture and the correction of imbalance and poor stance.

What happens when you visit an osteopath?

Your first visit to an osteopath might seem like any other medical consultation. The doctor will talk to you about your main complaint and probably question you about the nature of the pain, its onset, duration, and any aggravating and ameliorating factors. You will be asked about your general health and any major accidents or illnesses you have had in the past, all of which aid in the assessment of your individual needs.

The osteopath will then examine your spine and other joints. Usually you will be required to undress, because an important part of

osteopathic diagnosis involves feeling for texture and temperature changes on the skin, as well as pressing and moving—palpation—of the bones and muscles to identify problems.

The diagnosis often blends into treatment as the doctor gently feels the muscles or rocks the joints to test their flexibility. Initially, treatment focuses on stiffened or overstretched muscles, especially near the areas where they are attached to bones. Gentle easing of restricted joints and osteopathic adjustments may be carried out. For this an osteopath may place you in a position that isolates the affected joint, using your arms, legs, or trunk as leverage. A gentle thrust then painlessly releases the joint, often with an audible click or crackle.

What conditions can be improved with osteopathy?

Neck and back pain and injuries can be helped, particularly injuries to the joints, such as the shoulders and backbone. Other joint problems—for example in the hips, knees, and ankles—can also be treated, as well as arthritis and rheumatism. Migraine and other headaches and facial neuralgia can also be relieved by osteopathic treatment.

Are there any contraindications?

In the hands of a qualified practitioner, osteopathy is an extremely safe form of treatment. A qualified osteopath is competent in medical diagnosis and will arrange X-rays or referral to your primary-care doctor

Origins

Andrew Taylor Still (1828–1917) was a frontier doctor in the United States who became disillusioned with conventional medicine after the death of two of his children from meningitis. He studied magnetic healing and bonesetting, using this knowledge to build on his new theory of osteopathy. Manipulation could, Still decided, restore balance and cure illness because the structure of the bones and posture play an important role in health. He launched osteopathy in 1874 and founded the first school for practitioners in 1892 in Kirksville, Missouri.

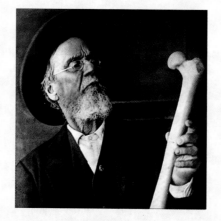

ANDREW TAYLOR STILL
A.T. Still viewed the body as a machine, with each part affecting the functioning of all the other parts. He concluded that illness arises when the body's structure slips out of alignment, preventing the parts from interacting smoothly.

if there is any cause for concern. There are no side effects from properly conducted osteopathic treatment, but occasionally some soreness may be felt after the initial examination or treatment, which usually goes away after a few days. If in doubt about any post-treatment discomfort, speak to your osteopath, who will be able to explain what is happening and suggest drug-free ways of relieving it.

How often and for how long will I need to be treated?

The frequency of sessions depends on how severe your pain is and how it can best be treated. For many conditions your osteopath may give two or three treatments a week. As the condition improves, this schedule will be reduced to once a week.

Weekly treatment is given initially for most long-lasting chronic disorders, the frequency gradually being reduced to fortnightly or monthly visits as you progress to more comfort and self-sufficiency.

What is the difference between osteopathy and chiropractic?

The objectives of osteopathy and chiropractic are very similar—to restore musculoskeletal integrity and thereby improve the balance and

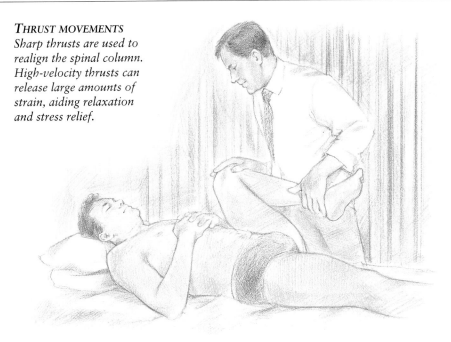

*THRUST MOVEMENTS
Sharp thrusts are used to realign the spinal column. High-velocity thrusts can release large amounts of strain, aiding relaxation and stress relief.*

health of the body as a whole. To achieve these aims chiropractors focus on the spinal column and the individual vertebral segments, whereas osteopaths also target muscles and other soft tissues, plus joints and ligaments, with their treatment (including those of the skull in the case of practitioners using cranial osteopathy).

In practice there is much overlap in the way that the two professions treat their patients, but there are some differences in technique. For

instance, osteopaths tend to use the limbs and trunk of the patient to provide leverage in making their adjustments, whereas chiropractors favor a high-velocity thrust directly on individual vertebral segments.

Finally, properly qualified osteopaths will have the letters D.O. (doctor of osteopathic medicine) after their name. This means that they have trained at one of the accredited schools of osteopathy in the United States and have also done a medical residency in a hospital.

AFTER AN OSTEOPATHIC SESSION

A brisk walk will help your body to settle after osteopathic treatment. A good all-round exercise, walking helps you burn off fat, tone muscles, and breathe properly. At the same time it does not put undue strain on any of your bones, joints, or muscles. To gain the most benefit, walk for at least 20 minutes and make sure that you have good footwear and are dressed for the weather. Move briskly, taking deep breaths of air and maintaining a good posture. You may find that you can use the time to reflect on any problems you have; fresh air can often help you think more clearly.

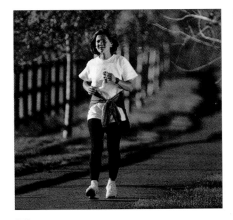

*WALKING FOR HEALTH
Walking is beneficial for mobility and muscular coordination. It aids normal body functions without straining you.*

BENEFITS OF WALKING

► *Improves blood circulation.*
► *Helps keep bones strong.*
► *Exercises the muscular system.*
► *Is great for the heart.*
► *Improves joint mobility.*
► *Is a good aerobic exercise.*
► *Has a low impact: will not damage your joints.*
► *Is excellent for body functions.*
► *Helps you lose excess fat.*
► *Has therapeutic qualities.*
► *Gives you time to think.*

CRANIOSACRAL THERAPY

CranioSacral therapy involves gentle manipulation of the skull. It eases migraines, other headaches, and tension and can be effective in treating stress and a range of mental disorders.

The sensitivity of the cranium to gentle manipulation has been realized only in recent times. Until well into this century, it was believed that the bones of the skull became fixed by the time a person reached 35 years of age, hindering advancements in the cranial field. Since the Second World War, it has been recognized that the skull continues to grow throughout life, and its condition can have a serious impact on both our physical health and mental state.

ORIGINS

In the early 20th century, Dr. William Sutherland, an osteopath, first realized the significance of the cranium in overall health and balance. He developed cranial osteopathy, a refined, hands-on technique used to detect and treat subtle disturbances in motion patterns in the skull, which may be symptomatic of certain disorders.

CranioSacral therapy formally emerged in the late 1970s, when John Upledger, an osteopath in the United States, set up a research team that uncovered new relationships between the cranium and the craniosacral system. From the results of this study he patented CranioSacral therapy.

PHILOSOPHY AND METHOD

The brain and spinal cord, which comprise the central nervous system, are surrounded by cerebrospinal fluid and membranes known as meninges. A malfunction or imbalance in this system can contribute to a number of general health disorders. Gentle massage of the head changes the pressure of the cerebrospinal fluid and meninges, rebalancing the central nervous system.

CranioSacral therapists, using a precise mapping of the skull, work particularly on the fine fissures that they describe as joints. The practice involves using very gentle bone manipulations, or palpations. To a large extent this therapy draws on the subtle sensings and intuition of the practitioner, a fact that concerns many mainstream physicians. Because some CranioSacral therapists lack training in anatomy and physiology, doctors fear that they may not recognize serious medical conditions.

PROBLEMS TREATED

CranioSacral therapy is used to treat children and adults for problems ranging from mood disorders to migraine, dyslexia, autism, stroke, epilepsy, multiple sclerosis, cerebral palsy, chronic pain, jaw problems such as temporomandibular joint disorder, and general stress disorders.

GENTLE TOUCH
CranioSacral practitioners draw both on knowledge acquired during training and on their own intuition to guide their gentle manipulations of the skull.

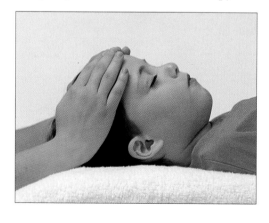

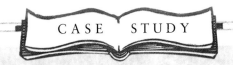

A Migraine Sufferer

Migraine headaches can strike at any moment, completely debilitating the sufferer and making work and normal routines very difficult. Some patients find that CranioSacral therapy can greatly reduce the severity of migraine by helping to rebalance the fluids in the head and spine, thus restoring them to health and allowing them to return to normal activity.

Joan, 52 years old, has a busy and stressful job as an administrator in a hospital. She has suffered from periodic migraines for the past seven or eight years, but recently they have been getting worse, especially since the death of her husband 10 months ago. She has had to take long stretches of time off from work, which she cannot afford to do. Her doctor has prescribed painkillers, but they have lost their effectiveness because she has been taking them often. They are also disrupting her ability to concentrate. The pain has caused her to be short-tempered frequently with colleagues, family members, and friends and to fear social activities. Her family is becoming increasingly concerned that she is isolating herself too much.

WHAT SHOULD JOAN DO?

Joan could consider trying an alternative approach such as CranioSacral therapy to deal with her migraines. The therapist will seek to detect and massage any abnormalities in the flow of her cerebrospinal fluid, which would alleviate the pain by dealing directly with its cause. In contrast, the painkillers she has been taking deal only with symptoms and thus are not a long-term solution. Joan needs also to recognize the emotional toll that her husband's death has taken and seek professional counseling or discuss her problems and feelings with family and friends. She should definitely make an effort to relax more and consider ways to make her job less stressful.

Action Plan

FAMILY
Try to recognize and express emotional pain and share it with family and close friends. Letting go can be healthier than trying to stay always in control.

WORK
Take some of the stress off the work situation by cutting down the hours and sharing some of the responsibilities.

LIFESTYLE
Use relaxation and simple self-massage techniques to improve circulation, relieve stress, and encourage feelings of well-being.

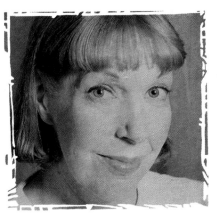

LIFESTYLE
Stress and lack of exercise can increase the likelihood of migraines.

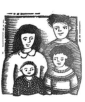

FAMILY
Bereavement increases emotional strain, opening the doors to ill health.

WORK
An overly stressful job is not good for health and exacerbates poor health conditions and migraines.

HOW THINGS TURNED OUT FOR JOAN

One of Joan's colleagues directed her to a CranioSacral therapist at a local clinic. After a 10-week course of treatment, her migraines cleared up and her general health improved dramatically. She now plays golf regularly for exercise. Joan also managed to have a long talk with her daughter, which has helped both of them to come to terms with the loss of a husband and father. Work is as demanding as ever, but Joan feels so much better that she is now taking it in stride.

CHIROPRACTIC

Chiropractic is the manipulation of the backbone to realign the vertebrae. This helps to restore proper functioning of the central nervous system and balance the energy of the body.

Chiropractic (from the Greek words *cheiro* and *praktikos*, meaning "done by hand") is now found everywhere in the world. In many countries, particularly in the West, it is the third largest medical profession, behind dentistry and orthodox medicine. This is particularly true in the United States, Canada, Australia, and New Zealand, where it has been adopted into mainstream health care.

ORIGINS

Chiropractic was founded in 1895 by Daniel David Palmer, a self-taught healer in the United States. A porter who worked in his building had become deaf following a back injury. By correcting the displacement of a vertebra in the man's spine, Palmer restored his hearing. Palmer theorized that it was the disruption of the central nervous system that had caused the hearing problem, and from this discovery he went on to develop the practice of chiropractic.

Behind the theory was his belief that the brain sends energy to every body organ along nerves that run through the spinal cord, and that displaced vertebrae can interfere with normal nerve transmission, thus causing health problems.

He founded the first chiropractic school and treatment center in Davenport, Iowa, in 1898 but left it in 1902 to spread the practice around North America. He died in 1913. His son, Bartlett Joshua Palmer, took over the chiropractic school at the age of 21 and was its president from 1906 until his death in 1961. Bartlett proclaimed chiropractic to the world, at one time even awarding mail-order degrees. Flamboyant and entrepreneurial, he also ran a printing press and launched a radio station within the college, the second commercial broadcasting station in the United States. An osteological museum of 10,000 spines was established under his direction.

TRAINING

A doctor of chiropractic (D.C.) in the United States must complete at least two years of undergraduate study and a four-year course at a chiropractic college. Some universities offer a bachelor's degree in chiropractic, after which graduate study at a chiropractic school is required. Practitioners must also pass a rigorous state board exam to be licensed in the state where they work.

Canadian chiropractors graduate from the Canadian Memorial Chiropractic College in Toronto or the Université du

CAUSES OF NERVE DISORDERS

Daniel David Palmer divided the causes of nerve disorders into five broad categories in order to simplify diagnosis and enable efficient treatment. The source of the problem is an important clue to finding the proper cure, and a chiropractor may ask many questions to get to the root of a problem.

Physical
Injury, surgery, malnutrition, and illness or disease, such as diabetes, can cause nerve problems.

Genetic
Various hereditary conditions, such as multiple sclerosis and muscular dystrophy, can disrupt nerve functioning.

Thermal
Staying out in the cold too long or taking a cold shower can lead to numbness and nerve dysfunction.

Causes of nerve disorders

Mental
Emotional breakdown, psychosomatic problems, drug abuse, anxiety, and stress can all cause nerve disorders.

Chemical
Man-made toxins, such as pesticides or industrial poisons, can impair the transmission of nerve impulses.

Québec in Trois-Rivières or from one of the U.S. colleges. Graduates of U.S. schools must pass special Canadian examinations in order to practice in one of the provinces. Treatment is covered by some government health insurance and many private health insurance plans in both the United States and Canada.

PHILOSOPHY AND METHOD

Chiropractic is based on the theory that when there is a misalignment of the spine, known as a subluxation, this affects the entire body—the central nervous system and the immune system.

Practitioners generally have one of two basic approaches. They adhere strictly to making adjustments—finding and eliminating subluxations—or they combine spinal adjustments with other therapies like heat treatment and counseling on nutrition and appropriate exercises. The first approach is called "straight," the second one, "mixed."

Like an orthodox physician, a chiropractor takes a medical history and performs an examination, the focus of which is usually to assess muscle strength or weakness and the range of spinal motion and joint mobility and to look for structural deformities or postural problems. Before giving any treatment, he or she will take X-rays of the spine to locate vertebral misalignments and areas of spinal stress and make certain there is no tumor or fracture, which would require referral to a physician.

The two most common adjustment methods are high-velocity thrusts and rotational thrusts. For the first, the patient lies on a special table with sections that drop or move slightly downward as adjustments are made. For the second, the patient lies with the upper body twisted sideways to the limit of its normal movement, and the practitioner applies a short, fast thrust to the spine.

PROBLEMS TREATED

Chiropractic is particularly effective for dealing with back and neck pain due to various causes. It can also be useful for treating migraines and other headaches, sciatica, shoulder pain, tennis elbow, and pains in a leg, hand, foot, or wrist.

By keeping the system in balance, chiropractic is sometimes useful as a preventive therapy. (In one study, removal of nerve blockage significantly enhanced athletes' agility, power, balance, and speed.) It may

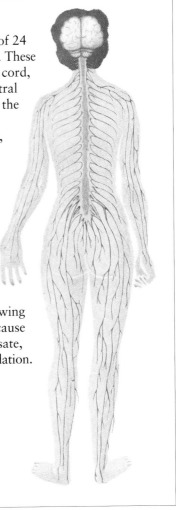

THE NERVOUS SYSTEM

The backbone, or spine, is made up of 24 small, interlinked bones, or vertebrae. These form a chain that protects the spinal cord, which, with the brain, forms the central nervous system. Nerves extend from the vertebrae to each part of the body, connecting the backbone to each bone, muscle, and organ in the entire body. These nerves are used to convey messages such as pain and touch to and from the brain.

If the spine is in any way out of balance, it will cause a malfunction in the nervous system. This may affect the transmission of nerve signals to and from the brain and lead to illness or pain or more subtle problems like the slowing of the function of an organ. It may cause another part of the body to compensate, leading to fatigue and general degradation.

HOW WE FEEL TOUCH
When your fingers touch something, the feeling is picked up by the nerves and sent to the brain, where it is registered. The brain decides on a response, which is sent back via the nervous system to the hand.

be beneficial, too, for treating stress and trauma. Despite continuing doubts by some orthodox doctors, chiropractic has many devoted followers who have found relief with it when other approaches have failed. There is also some research that shows it to be effective in lowering blood pressure.

CONTRAINDICATIONS

Certain manipulations carry some risk, and you may be asked to sign a waiver. Patients who have osteoporosis and other disorders characterized by weak or brittle bones should avoid chiropractic, otherwise, there are few circumstances for which it should not be used. Treatment for the weak or frail, however, must be less vigorous. A practitioner should discuss any risks or problems beforehand and adjust the program accordingly. Patients suffering from major disorders such as cancer, heart disease, or diabetes can be treated by a chiropractor but never as a substitute for traditional medical treatment.

PHYSIOTHERAPY

Encompassing a range of techniques, physiotherapy is now part of mainstream health care and plays an important role in pain relief and recovery from injuries and surgery.

PHYSIOTHERAPY AIDS RECOVERY

The various physiotherapy treatments work in different ways to improve health and mobility.

▶ *Hydrotherapy promotes the recovery of wasted muscle through exercise but without strain.*

▶ *Heat treatment dilates blood vessels to increase blood flow, improving the availability of oxygen and nutrients.*

▶ *Ice packs help reduce inflammation by constricting blood vessels and reducing blood flow.*

▶ *Massage relaxes joints and muscles to help restore flexibility.*

Physiotherapy aims to help relieve pain and speed the recovery of patients after injury or surgery. It has a scientific rather than a philosophical grounding and has therefore been more readily accepted by mainstream health care practitioners than other alternative therapies. It is widely available, and physiotherapy departments have been established in most hospitals. Many therapists have specialties in specific areas, such as orthopedics, gerontology, sports injuries, and pediatrics.

ORIGINS

The history of physiotherapy differs from that of osteopathy and chiropractic, in that it grew directly out of orthopedic medicine and has always been attached to orthodox health care. Hugh Owen Thomas founded orthopedic medicine in the late 19th century as a more conservative form of bonesetting that eschewed forceful joint manipulations. Physiotherapy was developed from this basis during the First World War by a team of nurses practicing massage. They initially called themselves the Society of Trained Masseuses, and this group later became the Chartered Society of Physiotherapy.

Patients were usually referred to physiotherapists by orthopedic specialists. They were treated with heat and massage and taught exercises that would restore proper functioning. Following the Second World War, orthopedic medicine developed alongside rheumatology departments in hospitals, and increasing use was made of physiotherapy, particularly after the development of ultrasound and electric-current techniques. Physiotherapy now plays a mainstream role in rehabilitation after surgery, injury, and

TYPES OF TREATMENT

Starting with basic massage and heat, physiotherapy has now incorporated a range of techniques for easing pain and aiding recovery. The practitioner decides which technique is appropriate for the treatment of a condition or disorder.

THERAPY	METHOD	PROBLEMS TREATED
Soft tissue massage	A range of muscle, joint, and soft-tissue massages and manipulations	Used for tense muscles, cramps, stress, and fatigue and to keep muscles active
Heat treatment	Use of a hot compress or heating lamp to warm the area and speed recovery	Good for torn muscles or ligaments, sprained joints, and osteoarthritis pains
Ultrasound treatment	Use of high-frequency sound waves to speed up healing	Helps soft-tissue injuries to recover, especially muscles and ligaments
Diathermy treatment	The use of high-frequency electric currents or microwaves to increase blood flow	Used for the recovery of soft tissue and to treat small cancerous tumors
Ice packs	Placing an ice pack over a wound or injury to cause blood to slow and to reduce swelling	Good instant relief for wounds and injuries; frequently used for sports injuries
Hydrotherapy	Using a pool for weight-free exercise; use of steam or water for injury relief	Used mostly for recovery from major injury or an operation to revive muscles

strokes, and many centers for physiotherapy are located in hospitals.

TRAINING

In the United States, practitioners must have completed four years of university study in physiotherapy, plus practical training, and met licensing requirements in the state where they practice. In Canada, physiotherapy is a provincially licensed, self-regulated profession. Practitioners must have a university degree in physiotherapy and have completed a clinical internship.

METHOD

Physiotherapists draw on a range of methods to aid the recovery of damaged tissue and relieve pain, employing them in various combinations. Two important aspects of treatment are therapeutic massage and exercise, both used to stretch muscles and improve joint mobility. Depending on a patient's condition, a therapist will manipulate him or her through various exercises or teach the patient how to do them at home.

Another approach, heat treatment, is used to promote recovery from an injury, such as a torn muscle, and relieve osteoarthritis, as heat is thought to stimulate the healing of tissues. Heat is administered through a hot compress, a dry heating pad, or a heating lamp that produces infrared rays.

Ultrasound, high-frequency sound waves, and diathermy, high-frequency electric currents or microwaves, may be used to speed healing of torn muscles and strained ligaments. Both are thought to stimulate blood flow and aid in soft-tissue recovery.

Ice packs are commonly employed also. Application of an ice pack to an injury reduces the flow of blood and stops swelling.

Another useful tool of the physiotherapist is hydrotherapy, the use of a swimming pool or whirlpool bath in which the patient can exercise without putting body weight on tender or weak muscles. It can also encompass a wide range of other water treatments, such as steam baths, flotation tanks, and high-pressure showers.

PROBLEMS TREATED

There are many problems that can be made better through physiotherapy; probably the most obvious are muscle and ligament injuries. Sports injuries, in particular, can be greatly helped by physiotherapy, especially

during the recovery period, when the treatment can improve muscle strength.

Physiotherapy departments in hospitals are often called on to help patients who are recovering from major surgery or those who have mobility problems following an injury or a stroke.

CONTRAINDICATIONS

There are no contraindications for physiotherapy generally, but some treatments should be avoided in certain circumstances. For example, anyone who has high blood pressure or heart trouble should not be given high-frequency treatments. If you are seeking treatment, the therapist will need to know full details of your state of health in order to decide which methods of therapy to use and which to avoid.

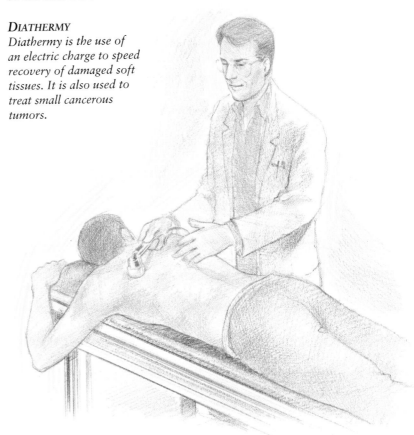

DIATHERMY
Diathermy is the use of an electric charge to speed recovery of damaged soft tissues. It is also used to treat small cancerous tumors.

Exercises in Water

Practitioners of all therapies advise backache sufferers to exercise in a swimming pool if possible. The body is supported by the water, which allows the joints and muscles to be moved and stretched without bearing the weight of the body.

SWIMMING FOR HEALTH

Swimming, one of the best forms of aerobic exercise, utilizes more muscles than almost any other sport and improves lung capacity. But its biggest advantage is that water supports the weight of the body, allowing muscles to be stretched and exercised without straining the bones and joints.

The following exercises are useful for everyone, not just people with back problems, because they move the joints and muscles, relax muscle tension, and make movement easier. Since the water sustains your weight, these exercises will not strain you at all; even the very frail can do them. All the stretches should be done near the wall of a pool at a depth where the side or the bar that you will be holding onto is positioned between your elbow and shoulder when you stand next to it.

EXERCISE 1

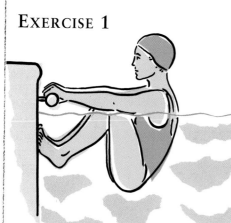

1 *In the pool, holding onto the edge or a bar with both hands, tuck your knees up between your elbows and touch the side of the pool with your toes.*

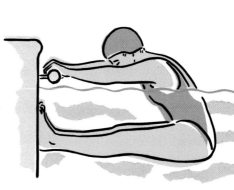

2 *Keep a firm grip on the pool edge or bar and push your feet flat against the wall, forcing your legs to straighten and pushing your body away. You will feel muscles stretching in your shoulders and back.*

EXERCISE 2

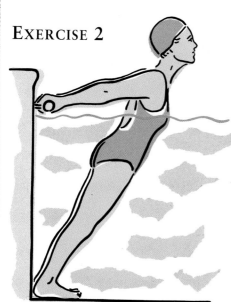

1 *Standing with your back to the wall of the pool, take hold of the edge or bar with both hands. Your feet should be flat on the floor, with heels right up against the wall.*

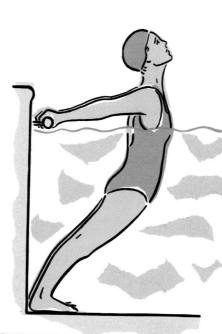

2 *Let your body fall forward, straightening your arms and allowing the water to take most of your weight. Push your pelvis forward and downward until you can feel the muscles stretch in your lower back and shoulder joints. Hold for as long as possible.*

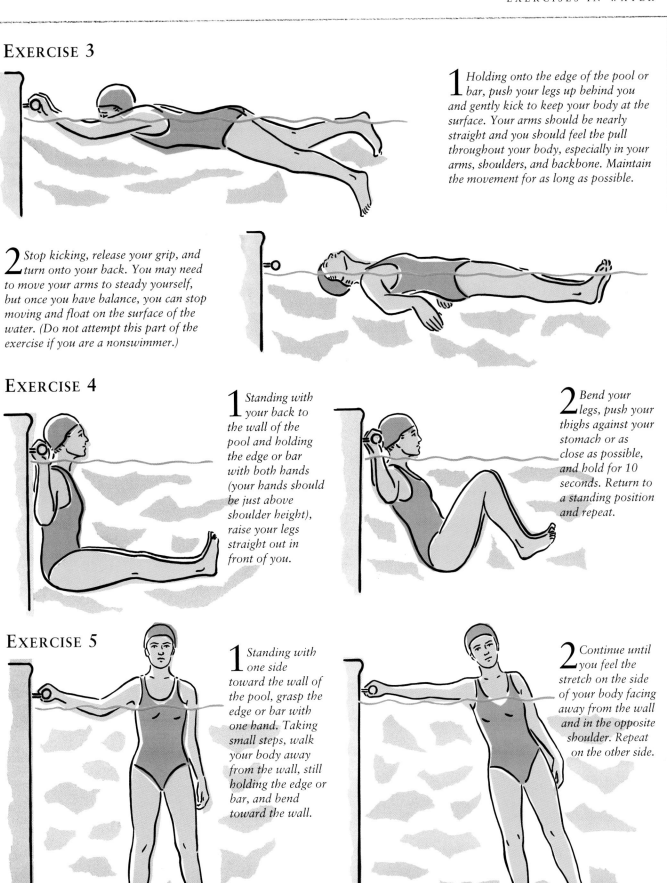

EXERCISE 3

1 Holding onto the edge of the pool or bar, push your legs up behind you and gently kick to keep your body at the surface. Your arms should be nearly straight and you should feel the pull throughout your body, especially in your arms, shoulders, and backbone. Maintain the movement for as long as possible.

2 Stop kicking, release your grip, and turn onto your back. You may need to move your arms to steady yourself, but once you have balance, you can stop moving and float on the surface of the water. (Do not attempt this part of the exercise if you are a nonswimmer.)

EXERCISE 4

1 Standing with your back to the wall of the pool and holding the edge or bar with both hands (your hands should be just above shoulder height), raise your legs straight out in front of you.

2 Bend your legs, push your thighs against your stomach or as close as possible, and hold for 10 seconds. Return to a standing position and repeat.

EXERCISE 5

1 Standing with one side toward the wall of the pool, grasp the edge or bar with one hand. Taking small steps, walk your body away from the wall, still holding the edge or bar, and bend toward the wall.

2 Continue until you feel the stretch on the side of your body facing away from the wall and in the opposite shoulder. Repeat on the other side.

METAMORPHIC TECHNIQUE

Combining the physical benefits of reflexology with a psychological approach all its own, metamorphic technique is a unique contribution to touch therapies.

Robert St. John founded this method in the 1960s. He first called it prenatal therapy, but it soon became known as metamorphic technique. It is based on the holistic idea that a small part of the body—the foot, for example—is representative of the whole person. By working on one small part, you can change and renew the whole self. The practitioners look upon themselves as catalysts in that they are the instruments through which individual patients are enabled to fulfill their true potential. There is a strong metaphysical undercurrent to the approach, with an emphasis on life and life force, change, and creation. Similes, such as a caterpillar metamorphosing into a butterfly or an acorn growing into an oak tree, are used to illustrate the potential that the individual possesses for transformation.

ORIGINS

In the 1960s Robert St. John, a naturopath, was increasingly dissatisfied with the treatments available for mentally handicapped children. He explored reflexology and went on to create his own charts, using intuition to map reflex points on the feet. He distinguished two basic patterns in human behavior: the afferent, which is inward moving, and the efferent, which is outward going. As extreme examples of these, he cited the autistic person as someone inward and pulling away from life, and the Down's syndrome person as outward and attracted to life.

TRAINING

Although there are a few specialized colleges, most practitioners of metamorphic technique are naturopaths or reflexologists who have taken additional courses or studied the technique on their own.

PHILOSOPHY AND METHOD

Robert St. John, who was aware of the psychological and emotional effects of reflexology, superimposed a psychological map onto the physical reflexology map of the foot. He deduced that the heel area corresponds to the base of the spine, the sexual organs, and the place of birth: he called this the mother

PRENATAL PATTERN

Before and during birth, a baby may experience a number of traumas that can affect health and emotional balance. Metamorphic technique aims to resolve these traumas by working through the nine-month gestation period. Practitioners believe that the prenatal period is reflected in a subtle line along each foot, which they work on thoroughly. There are similar lines on the hands and cranium, which they work on after completing the feet.

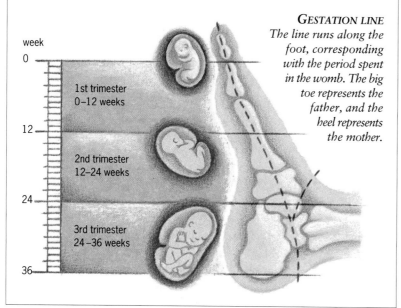

*GESTATION LINE
The line runs along the foot, corresponding with the period spent in the womb. The big toe represents the father, and the heel represents the mother.*

week
0

1st trimester
0–12 weeks

12

2nd trimester
12–24 weeks

24

3rd trimester
24–36 weeks

36

principle. He also believed that if there was a difficulty in the relationship with the mother, this would be apparent in blockages or imbalances present in the heel. He went on to seek the father principle, the external figure of authority and power, which he designated as the big toe area around the first joint.

Through intuition, St. John drew a time map between these two points, representing the nine-month period spent in the womb. (This the reason that St. John initially called his system prenatal therapy.) Metamorphists claim that by working on the various points between the toe and the heel they can affect the characteristics that make up the individual—the characteristics that were laid down in the womb. Practitioners of this technique also claim to look beyond the maps to find the life force itself. It is this life force, they believe, that can bring about a permanent change, or cure, in the patient.

A metamorphic technique session

The session will begin with the practitioner taking the right foot and gently touching the bone down the inside of the foot and across the ankle, using small, circular movements with the fingertips. The practitioner then takes the big toe in one hand and the heel in the other and works on both simultaneously. This procedure is repeated on the left foot. It is said that the feet represent energy and movement and, as each part is touched and massaged, old problems are dispersed, making way for new ideas and change.

The hands, representing action, and the head, representing thought, can be worked on in a similar way, with different points relating to the mother and father principles and affecting different aspects.

PROBLEMS TREATED

Practitioners of metamorphic technique do not try to treat particular symptoms but instead to help a person understand his or her deeper personality and psychological problems and to identify behavioral patterns that may be detrimental. They believe they can uncover and resolve emotional difficulties that have led to stress. They also claim that they can help people understand and break learned behavior patterns that contribute to long-standing health problems and that lead to ongoing personal or emotional troubles.

CONTRAINDICATIONS

This is a general therapy rather than a treatment for specific medical conditions. There are no contraindications to metamorphic technique, although it has been suggested that care should be taken with self-analysis, which might lead to a misdiagnosis that could have emotional or physical repercussions. Many doctors are concerned that there is danger in relying on techniques such as this, as they can potentially distract a patient from serious medical problems that may need more thorough medical treatment.

GINGER FOOT BATH

This foot bath is excellent for soothing and reviving tired and strained feet. The tea tree oil adds a strong disinfectant, which cleanses the feet thoroughly and helps to clear up infections and fungal conditions such as athlete's foot.

1 small onion	3 liters (6 quarts) hot water
1 clove garlic	25 g (1 oz) dried sage
3 cm (1 in) piece fresh gingerroot	25 g (1 oz) dried rosemary
	20 drops tea tree essential oil

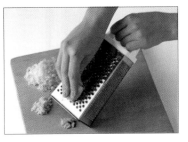

1 *Chop the onion and garlic finely and grate the gingerroot. Heat the water in a large saucepan and add the onion, garlic, gingerroot, and herbs. Simmer gently for 5 minutes.*

2 *Remove from the heat and allow to infuse for 10 minutes. Strain the liquid and leave to cool slightly—about 4 minutes. Add the tea tree oil and pour the liquid into a large bowl or shallow tub.*

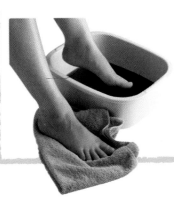

3 *Soak your feet for 20 minutes, covering them and the bowl with a towel to prevent the heat from escaping. Move your feet around from time to time to keep the mixture properly blended. Pat your feet dry, taking care to dry thoroughly between your toes.*

ROLFING

Rolfing involves therapeutic pummeling of the deeper layers of the body's connective tissues. Promoting relaxation, it is also renowned for its psychological and emotional benefits.

In the United States, between the world wars, Dr. Ida Rolf devised a therapy that was first known as Structural Integration and eventually as Rolfing. Using pressure and stretch techniques, she worked on the fasciae—connective tissues that join the muscles, bones, and organs—to reorganize and balance the body.

ORIGINS

Rolfing is based on the mind-body link and life energy. Dr. Ida Rolf, a leading biochemist, believed that there are two separate energies that affect the body—gravity and the sun—and the beneficial qualities of these energies can be felt only when the fasciae are in complete balance.

It wasn't until the 1950s that Structural Integration started to become better known, when Ida Rolf presented her work to osteopaths and chiropractors in the United States, Canada, and the United Kingdom. Since then, osteopathy and chiropractic have been

DR. IDA ROLF
Known for her warmth and kindness, Dr. Ida Rolf promoted fascia relaxation through Rolfing for everyone, from babies to the elderly.

greatly influenced by Rolfing, and many other touch therapists now employ an element of Rolfing in their techniques.

Rolfing became popular during the 1960s when New Age therapies arose along with the relaxation of strict social codes and a more critical attitude toward conventional medicine. Rolfing was discovered to release repressed and inhibited emotional tensions from the muscles in the body, and it became a popular therapy for people who wanted to discover more about themselves.

TRAINING

Professional training courses are hard to find outside the United States, where a number of colleges offer three- or four-year courses leading to a professional qualification. There are, however, many informal classes available, designed for people who wish to massage their friends and learn more about the Rolfing philosophy.

PHILOSOPHY AND METHOD

Dr. Rolf claimed that the role of the fasciae in the body was ignored by modern medicine. The fasciae are an all-encompassing

TEN SESSIONS OF ROLFING

Typically, a complete Rolfing treatment will consist of 10 hour-long sessions spread over a number of weeks; commonly, people will have one or two sessions every week. Each session focuses on a set of muscles and joints and the surrounding fasciae, starting with the outer muscles and working to the deeper muscles. A complete 10-week course will cover every aspect of the body thoroughly.

The first session works on relaxing the fasciae in the hands and feet, restoring them to an optimum condition.

The early sessions (two to four) loosen fasciae in the arms and legs, improving their flexibility and muscles.

The middle sessions (five to seven) work deeply on the inner organs, particularly in the abdominal region.

The later sessions (eight to ten) concentrate on the back, the shoulders, and postural problems.

A Stressed Executive

Focusing exclusively on your working life can lead to excessive stress and put your health at risk, taking an emotional toll and detracting from your enjoyment of life. Rolfing therapy can help you relax, allowing you to consider your broader personal needs and perhaps giving you access to previously hidden emotions and problems.

Henry is 36 years old and constantly under pressure. His career as a highly motivated sales executive is very important to him, but his long and hectic working hours have led to bad eating habits and quite high levels of smoking and drinking. He was recently upset to learn that he has a stomach ulcer, and he realized, reluctantly, that he is suffering from severe stress. His family is worried because he doesn't socialize, except with work colleagues, and has not had a steady girlfriend for some time now. Privately, he finds it difficult to relax in a sexual relationship. The idea of being close to or intimate with someone frightens him, and he attempts to persuade himself that he is better off without a partner.

WHAT SHOULD HENRY DO?

Henry should regularly take some time away from work for exercise and relaxation. During these periods he should not even think about his job but consider instead his other needs and goals. A good massage therapy such as Rolfing would help ease the tensions that have built up and bring his mind back in touch with his body, allowing him to listen to its needs and feel more comfortable with accepting pleasure and relief. This could help him address his needs and fears concerning sex and question his attitudes and anxieties about intimate relationships. He would feel better, too, if he were to drink and smoke less and pay more attention to his diet.

Action Plan

LIFESTYLE
Take time out to relax properly. Meditation, t'ai chi, or some stretching exercises may help. Use this time to consider personal needs and goals outside of work.

DIET
Plan to eat regular, healthy meals and cut down on smoking and drinking. Finding a new hobby may help to break old drinking and social habits.

SEX LIFE
Give relationships a chance; taking things slowly might help to change old attitudes.

DIET
A poor diet and high alcohol intake leads to a lowered immune function, making you more susceptible to illness.

SEX LIFE
Shutting yourself off from working at a relationship will not make your physical and emotional needs disappear, and it can lead to stress and depression.

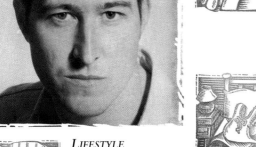

LIFESTYLE
Focusing on work to the exclusion of other aspects of life leads to physical imbalance and undue stress.

HOW THINGS TURNED OUT FOR HENRY

Every Saturday morning, for nearly three months, Henry had a Rolfing session. As well as finding it relaxing, he talked through a lot of his problems with the practitioner. This helped him place his work in perspective and enjoy his free time more. He has improved his eating habits and cut down on smoking and drinking, with the result that his ulcer has improved. He has joined a sports club and through this has met a new girlfriend.

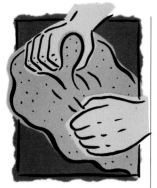

IMPROVING YOUR TOUCH

Making bread can be a relaxing and calming pastime, releasing the day's stress and allowing creativity to flow. It is also good for your hands, as it requires a keen sense of touch. Many professional bakers can use touch alone to judge the right consistency of the dough.

envelope, a continuous web of thin, elastic, connective tissue that binds the body parts together. Stretching, separating, and relaxing all the fasciae through massage can greatly improve health and mobility and affect both the emotional and physical states of being. Often the massage must be deep and penetrating to reach the inner layers of fasciae. Some people find Rolfing painful, and many practitioners make few concessions to lighten the regimen because it is meant to tackle deep tensions.

Rolfing is usually carried out in a program of 10 one-hour sessions. During the first few treatments the focus is on the limbs; after this the therapist works toward the backbone. Loosening the tissue involves using the fingers, thumbs, hands, and elbows to work into the joints, ligaments, and connective tissues, pummeling the tissues apart. Especially important areas are the ankles and wrists, the shoulders and neck, the diaphragm, the hips, and the backbone. Other areas of injury, stress, or tension are also worked on thoroughly, although the practitioner will take care not to disrupt any natural healing processes that may be taking place throughout the body.

PROBLEMS TREATED

Rolfing is not used for any specific problem: it is a general therapy to help someone become balanced both physically and psychologically. If you feel out of harmony with yourself or feel the need for emotional stress relief, Rolfing could be appropriate and may offer tremendous release.

CONTRAINDICATIONS

Rolfing should be used for general health and therapeutic purposes and must not replace conventional health care. The only contraindications are for those who have physical injuries or skin problems.

CONVENTIONAL OPINION

Rolfing is generally considered a pleasant means of relaxing both the mind and the body. However, because its mind-body approach does not work on a conventional scientific basis, those with specific conditions are advised to see a doctor.

HELLERWORK

Similar to Rolfing, Hellerwork involves the relaxing of the fasciae, or connective tissues, in order to improve the mind-body relationship. It was created in 1978 by Joseph Heller, a former U.S. aerospace engineer, to help patients break away from set patterns of moving, thinking, and feeling. Hellerwork helps them to balance their own lives and adapt to change.

The therapy utilizes massage, manipulation, movement, and discussion. It is primarily aimed at getting rid of stress and tension by improving the body's structure and functioning and returning it to a more relaxed and youthful natural state.

It is divided into three distinct parts: body work, movement, and dialogue. These are treated separately, although they are recognized as linking parts of the whole. Dialogue is particularly stressed in Hellerwork, with the practitioner assuming a counselor's role. Joseph Heller saw the need for the release of emotional and mental tensions as well as physical ones. He emphasized that the way to full health was to question your belief systems. He personally believed that we all need to challenge our roles and behavior patterns in order to come to terms with our true needs and goals. In his view, this was the best path to health and complete personal fulfillment.

HELLERWORK

Joseph Heller was eager that his therapy not be limited to dealing with only one side of a person's life. He split it into three sections: body work, movement, and dialogue. This reflects the holistic nature of the therapy and Joseph Heller's belief that the physical body is closely linked to the emotions.

MOVEMENT
The patient is taught how to walk, sit, stand, and move in order to retain freedom of movement.

DIALOGUE
This is a discussion concerning how established belief patterns affect the patient's body.

BODY WORK
This involves the manipulation and massage of the body to stretch and relax the fasciae.

C H A P T E R 4

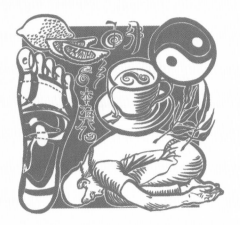

ENERGY REBALANCING THERAPIES

Energy is the basis of all life, and at the heart of the therapies in this chapter is the belief that the free flow of energy is essential to good health. The modern environment puts enormous pressure on our body systems and rhythms, often distorting or blocking our vitality. These therapies aim to clear any blockages, restoring balance to the energy systems within us and promoting harmony with the outside world.

ACUPRESSURE AND TUINA

Acupressure, the art of balancing body energy, can effectively relieve many common ailments. Tuina is a massage therapy based on acupressure points and whole-body balance.

Acupressure has been deeply embedded in Eastern medicine for many thousands of years, used both as a folk remedy and by traditional doctors. When it fell out of favor as part of medical practice, many forms were kept alive as home remedies, the wisdom being passed down from generation to generation. It is now gradually being readopted by professional doctors in the East as they realize its benefits as a natural healing system. Practiced throughout Asia, it is particularly popular in China, Japan, Korea, Tibet, Thailand, India, and the Philippines.

Tuina is a traditional Chinese system of massage that includes soft-tissue techniques and manipulations. It achieves remarkable results by working on the energy channels, or meridians, and their acupressure points. Traditional Tuina involves an extensive range of techniques, but a narrower range is often applied in Europe and North America. Though it is used primarily to redress energy imbalances and restore general health, specific conditions can be treated, particularly stress-related disorders and problems with self-confidence, depression, and anxiety.

ORIGINS

About 5,000 years ago, possibly in India, a systematized and intelligent approach to pressure points was first developed, and the instinct of touch became a skill. These healing skills were based on putting pressure on specific energy points to balance the body's energy, or qi (pronounced chee). Knowledge of pressure points gradually spread throughout Asia, often in connection with the spread of Buddhism by monks, with each culture putting its own stamp on the system, adapting it to the local culture and beliefs.

The background philosophy to acupressure is the same as that of traditional Chinese medicine. Whereas Western medicine aims to isolate the factors responsible for illness or disease and eradicate them, the Eastern approach concerns itself with the balance and flow of energies in the body. It is a philosophy that stresses the relationship between our inner condition and the outer

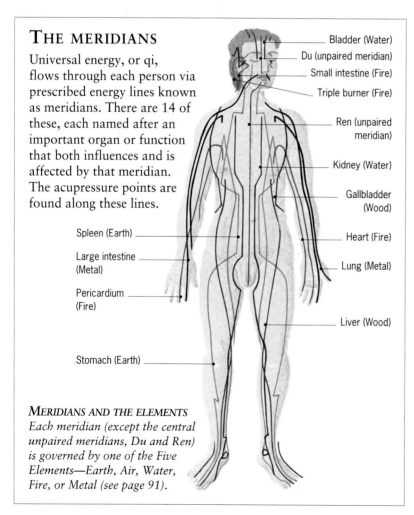

THE MERIDIANS

Universal energy, or qi, flows through each person via prescribed energy lines known as meridians. There are 14 of these, each named after an important organ or function that both influences and is affected by that meridian. The acupressure points are found along these lines.

Bladder (Water)
Du (unpaired meridian)
Small intestine (Fire)
Triple burner (Fire)
Ren (unpaired meridian)
Kidney (Water)
Gallbladder (Wood)
Heart (Fire)
Lung (Metal)
Liver (Wood)

Spleen (Earth)
Large intestine (Metal)
Pericardium (Fire)
Stomach (Earth)

MERIDIANS AND THE ELEMENTS
Each meridian (except the central unpaired meridians, Du and Ren) is governed by one of the Five Elements—Earth, Air, Water, Fire, or Metal (see page 91).

YIN AND YANG

According to traditional Chinese medicine, the whole universe originated from a unified source known as the Tao, which is present in everything. The Tao created two opposite forces—yin and yang—that are present in everything and are incomplete without each other. Each has opposing characteristics (see below) that work together to form the whole. It is the attraction between yin and yang that creates the movement of universal energy, and meridian therapies attempt to balance these forces to release energy blockages and improve energy flow.

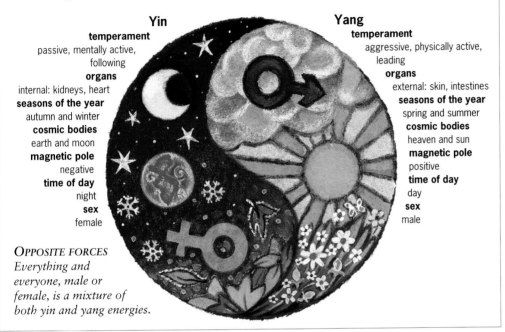

Yin
temperament
passive, mentally active, following
organs
internal: kidneys, heart
seasons of the year
autumn and winter
cosmic bodies
earth and moon
magnetic pole
negative
time of day
night
sex
female

Yang
temperament
aggressive, physically active, leading
organs
external: skin, intestines
seasons of the year
spring and summer
cosmic bodies
heaven and sun
magnetic pole
positive
time of day
day
sex
male

OPPOSITE FORCES
Everything and everyone, male or female, is a mixture of both yin and yang energies.

environment. We are seen to be affected by all things physical: weather, sounds, seasons, and colors. The aim is to bring all these factors into harmonious balance.

TRAINING

Acupressure is usually practiced in combination with Tuina or another therapy such as applied kinesiology (see page 86) or shiatsu (see page 90). At one time, a therapist would learn the skills from an older professional, possibly a family member, although today training has become more formal.

DID YOU KNOW?

According to Chinese myth, acupressure originated among a band of giants known as the sons of the reflected light. Highly developed spiritual beings standing seven feet tall, the sons were able to perceive the meridians and acupressure points. They healed by directing their own energy in a way that would correct imbalances.

PHILOSOPHY AND METHOD

Acupressure is one of several strands of traditional Chinese medicine (others include acupuncture, Chinese herbalism, and Tuina) and heals by balancing the flow of life energy, or qi. This is achieved by direct pressure with fingers or thumbs on recognized acupressure points along the energy channels, or meridians. The points are identified by their meridian and a number that indicates the position on the meridian line. Acupressure points are located where the meridians pass close to the surface of the body; at these spots the energy is open to influence.

Depending on the diagnosis, the practitioner might strengthen, calm, or disperse the passing life current. The idea is to restore or maintain a balance between the vigorous yang energy and the restraining yin. The two forces cannot exist without each other. Therefore, to increase your energy, you must absorb both yin and yang in equal proportions from your environment. When either yin or yang is stifled or blocked, the overall energy will be reduced,

Acupressure points for special problems

Some common problems can be relieved by putting firm, constant pressure on easy-to-find acupressure points. Keep your thumb or a fingertip on the point for a couple of minutes or more (up to 4) for the best effect.

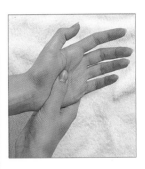

RESTLESSNESS
For insomnia, a restless or disturbed mind, or heart problems, press acupressure point Pericardium 8 for 2 minutes. It is located in the middle of the palm, straight down from the middle finger.

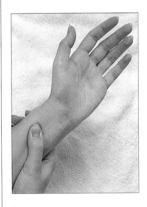

PAIN AND NAUSEA
One of the most powerful points, Pericardium 6 can help relieve motion sickness, pain, insomnia, and emotional anxiety. It is located on the underside of the arm, three finger widths from the wrist, between the two large tendons.

exposing the body to illness, fatigue, and generally poor health. The traditional Chinese medicine system emphasizes the need to release energy blocks through massage, herbal remedies, and healthy eating, and to maximize the absorption of yin and yang energies from external sources. For example, one could climb a mountain or do martial arts for more yang, or try decorative arts or similarly creative activities for more yin. Stimulation of acupressure points can clear the channels to increase the energies of both yin and yang forces, boosting the all-round vital energy.

SOOTHING EYE TONIC

This is an excellent treatment for relaxing sore or tired eyes; the chamomile acts as a skin softener, the witch hazel as a healer and mild antiseptic, and the frankincense as a soothing relaxant.

30 ml (2 tbsp) chamomile tea   5 ml (1 tsp) castor oil
30 ml (2 tbsp) witch hazel   2 drops frankincense oil

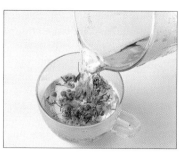 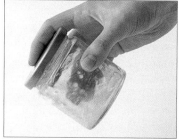

1 *Make the chamomile tea by infusing 2 tsp of dried chamomile flowers or 1 herbal tea bag in a cup of boiling water. Allow to cool and remove the herbs.*

2 *Mix 30 ml (2 tbsp) of the tea with the witch hazel in a screw-top jar. Add the castor oil and frankincense, replace the top tightly, and shake well.*

3 *Dip cotton eye pads or a clean face cloth into the liquid and soak thoroughly. Squeeze out any excess moisture, lie down, and place the pads over your closed eyes and forehead for at least 15 minutes. Relax and feel the healing tingle of the witch hazel.*

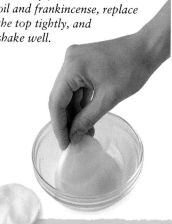

How to apply acupressure

There are three sorts of pressure that can be applied, according to the nature and severity of a problem. It is often best to start with a gentle, dispersing pressure and move toward more intense pressure if required, pressing each point for no more than four minutes.

Dispersing is a gentle, circular motion prescribed by the thumb or fingertip. This encourages the blocked energy to move, easing out tensions and restrictions.

Tonifying is achieved by stationary, firm pressure with thumb or fingertip perpendicular to the chosen point. This is generally done for two minutes to strengthen weak qi.

Calming is achieved by lightly covering the point with the palm or gently stroking the point with the fingers. Again, two minutes is usually sufficient to settle overactive energy.

PROBLEMS TREATED

Acupressure aims to redress imbalances and blockages found in the patient, and many problems or conditions can be treated by stimulating specific acupressure points or a number of points simultaneously. By increasing vitality, acupressure helps a patient overcome external symptoms, whether great or small. Acupressure alone is probably best suited to more minor ailments and home treatments, and Tuina for more complicated and thorough treatments. Acupressure is also ideally suited as a preventative treatment, which is, to a great extent, how it was originally intended.

CONTRAINDICATIONS

Acupressure and Tuina are fundamentally very safe. Rashes, boils, and varicose veins should be avoided, and there are a few pressure points to avoid if you have high blood pressure or if you are pregnant, so you must inform the practitioner beforehand.

CONVENTIONAL OPINION

Many doctors are happy to endorse a system such as acupressure that encourages treatment within the home for minor ailments. If symptoms do not clear up quickly, however, it's important to seek professional advice, in case the complaint is a serious one. Acupuncture, using needles instead of finger pressure, is popular with an increasing number of Western doctors who have come to understand the principles involved and recognize its effectiveness.

A Depressed Musician

Depression can be caused by a number of physical and emotional problems, although it usually reflects an imbalance in the sufferer that can become a vicious circle of uneasy emotions and hopelessness. Many energy balancing therapies can help ease depression, particularly Tuina, which focuses on releasing energy blocks and restoring balance and a sense of well-being.

Stephen, who is 28 years old, has been suffering from depression since his partner left him a year ago, making him feel both emotionally and sexually inadequate. He is having difficulty finding regular employment, and his financial situation is a constant worry. He has not been eating properly, has been sleeping badly, and now has skin problems and bad headaches. With his self-confidence at a low ebb, he has become reclusive and cynical about relationships. Fretting about his future as a musician and his failure at relationships has depressed him further, leading to a vicious circle of fear and self-doubt. A friend has suggested that he try some kind of stress-reducing therapy such as Tuina.

WHAT SHOULD STEPHEN DO?

Stephen would benefit from measures that can help him become more positive about life. Treated with an energy rebalancing therapy such as Tuina, he would feel better about himself and get back in touch with his needs, both physical and emotional. It would also help him relax so that he felt calmer and ready to explore the reasons for his depression. He may need to change some aspects of his lifestyle and begin to focus on what he really wants from life instead of dwelling on his current problems. He also should consider his future and realize that he would be happier if he put the past behind him and cleared the way for something new, different, and possibly exciting.

Action Plan

EATING HABITS
Maintain a balanced and healthy diet, trying not to skip meals. Cut down on caffeine and alcohol consumption to improve sleeping.

SEX LIFE
Don't ignore sexual and emotional needs. Meet new people and give relationships a chance. Stop dwelling on the past.

EMOTIONAL HEALTH
Put time aside to try to understand and resolve problems and restore emotional balance and self-confidence. Think positively and change your approach to life.

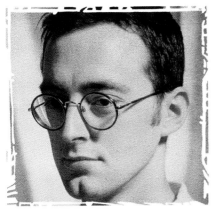

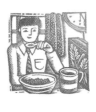

EATING HABITS
An unbalanced diet can lead to skin problems and poor health and cause depression and other psychological disorders as well.

SEX LIFE
Difficulties in accepting rejection from someone you love can prevent you from letting new people into your life, leaving you unfulfilled and depressed.

EMOTIONAL HEALTH
Dwelling on difficult emotional situations without working them through can create a downward spiral of depression.

HOW THINGS TURNED OUT FOR STEPHEN

After a course of Tuina, Stephen started to relax and became aware that his stress and anxiety were holding him back. He studied music therapy and found work as a therapist, using his skills to help disabled children express themselves through music. This brought him into contact with more people and improved his social life. His skin problems and headaches also cleared up, helped by a better sleeping routine and diet.

REFLEXOLOGY

The healing potential of reflexology is based on the theory that the body's energy channels can be unblocked, stimulated, and revitalized through sensitive reflex points on the feet.

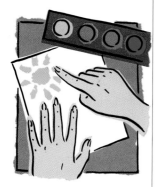

IMPROVING YOUR TOUCH

Dip your fingers into some paints and discover your feeling for art. The way that you use both the paint and the paper will be based on the way that your fingers feel the materials. Spend a little time considering the textures and touch sensations. It not only can help you improve your sense of touch but can also be highly relaxing, therapeutic, and fun.

ANCIENT FOOT THERAPY
The art of both the ancient Egyptians and North American Indians depicts the therapeutic use of foot massage.

Reflexology is not a new science but is really a 20th-century refinement of ancient wisdom that was largely ignored for 5,000 years before it resurfaced in the West. Reflexologists tend to think that its origins lie in traditional Chinese medicine, but direct evidence for this is hard to find. Research shows that many similar foot techniques were used in other cultures, for example, by the ancient Egyptians, some African tribes, and Native Americans.

ORIGINS

Reflexology's rediscovery, which occurred in the United States, was the combined result of the work of two people, Dr. William Fitzgerald and Eunice Ingham. In the early 1920s Dr. Fitzgerald, an ear, nose, and throat specialist, noticed that when some patients were in pain or anxious, they would clutch parts of their feet. He found that pressure on one part of the foot anesthetized the ear, allowing him to do minor surgery.

After extensive research and experimentation, he divided the body into 10 zones, each with a bioelectrical energy reflex point on the hands and feet. Fitzgerald recognized that manipulating these reflex points would alter the vital flow of energy within the corresponding body part and restore health.

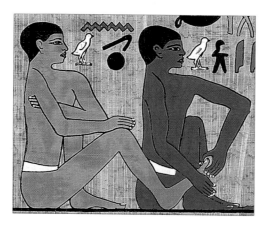

Fitzgerald's work, with assistance by his colleague Dr. Edwin Bowers, generated as much scorn as it did interest, and he was unable to launch the technique successfully. Eventually it was a nurse working for Dr. Bowers, Eunice Ingham, who completed development of the therapy. She reworked Fitzgerald's ideas and developed them into the more intricate system that we know today. An English nurse, Doreen Bayley, met Eunice Ingham and subsequently spread the practice of reflexology across Europe.

TRAINING

The International Institute of Reflexologists has established professional standards of education and teaching practices based on the Ingham methods. It certifies practitioners and provides referrals worldwide. The Reflexology Association of Canada, which has its own schooling and curricula, provides referrals for certified members in Canada.

PHILOSOPHY AND METHOD

Reflexology is based on vitalizing and clearing the energy pathways that run through the body and link the organs and other body parts. Reflexologists believe that the body and its workings are mirrored on the foot in the form of reflex points. This is known as microcosmic representation—the whole represented in the part. Massaging the reflex points unblocks universal life energy and activates the body's own healing powers. It works by stimulating, calming, and balancing energy flow through the foot and thereby throughout the whole body.

Tension relief

Stress and negative emotions restrict the flow of energy around the body. It is claimed that this lays the foundation for about 70 percent of all disorders. Under stress, the healthy blood and nerve supply to organs is constricted, which starves the tissues and organs and leads to a rise in toxins and an increased risk of illness.

Relaxation is the key word during treatment. Typically a session starts with a familiarizing and relaxing diagnostic foot massage and lasts about an hour. Both feet are thoroughly worked on in an unhurried fashion. Treatment can be somewhat painful at times, but this is always carefully monitored by the practitioner. Often a couple of treatments per week are recommended. Symptoms usually diminish after three or four treatments, although this will depend on many other factors. It is beneficial to carry on treatment after an illness in order to consolidate the healing process.

PROBLEMS TREATED

Good reflexologists can help improve a wide range of conditions. This is largely because treatment affects a person as a whole, raising inner vitality, and it is this raised vitality that moves a patient more quickly back to health. Stress-related conditions respond well to reflexology, as do digestive troubles, physical aches and pains, migraines and other headaches, menstrual complaints, and sinus and throat troubles.

CONTRAINDICATIONS

Responsible reflexology is never completely contraindicated, but because it is deceptively powerful, it needs to be used with extreme care in conditions that are associated with delicate metabolic balance. These would include pregnancy, diabetes, thyroid conditions, and heart disorders.

CONVENTIONAL OPINION

As long as no exaggerated claims are made, doctors are tolerant of reflexology, feeling that the associated stress reduction can benefit their patients and help them deal with minor complaints. However, the theory is backed with relatively little research and cannot be justified as therapy for any serious medical condition.

Home reflexology
Practicing reflexology at home can be fun and relaxing, although it usually takes time before you can give an effective treatment. Work your way from toes to heels, always treating the whole foot, not just one particular area.

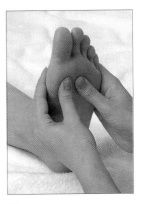

HEART REFLEX POINTS
This point on the ball of the foot corresponds to the heart, helping to boost good health.

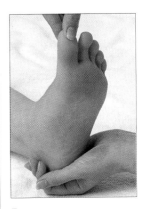

BRAIN REFLEX POINTS
This point on the end of the big toe is linked to the vitality of the mind.

REFLEXOLOGY MAP

The reflexology map was first drawn up by Dr. William Fitzgerald, and later refined by Eunice Ingham. The links between different parts of the body and points on the feet were worked out in detailed experiments, observing nerve and muscle reactions and the effects on body functioning and emotional well-being.

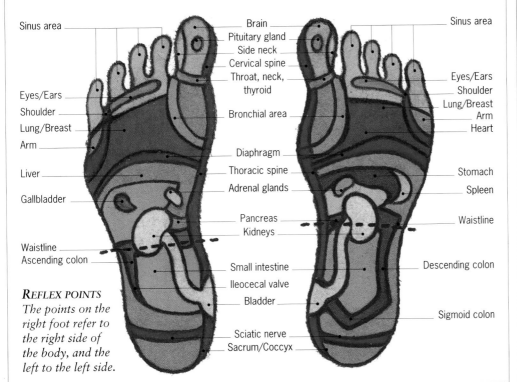

Sinus area · Brain · Pituitary gland · Side neck · Cervical spine · Throat, neck, thyroid · Sinus area · Eyes/Ears · Shoulder · Eyes/Ears · Shoulder · Lung/Breast · Arm · Lung/Breast · Arm · Bronchial area · Heart · Liver · Diaphragm · Thoracic spine · Adrenal glands · Stomach · Spleen · Gallbladder · Pancreas · Kidneys · Waistline · Waistline · Ascending colon · Descending colon · Small intestine · Ileocecal valve · Bladder · Sigmoid colon · Sciatic nerve · Sacrum/Coccyx

REFLEX POINTS
The points on the right foot refer to the right side of the body, and the left to the left side.

APPLIED KINESIOLOGY

Applied kinesiology aims to identify health problems by testing muscle reactions. Through this technique, it is the body itself that indicates the cause of imbalances and other problems.

THE BODY'S SYSTEMS

There are five bodily systems to be considered when muscle testing. These should be in balance and must be assessed together, as each affects and is affected by the others.

▶ *The nervous system*
▶ *The lymphatic system*
▶ *The vascular system*
▶ *The cerebrospinal system*
▶ *The acupressure-meridian system*

Acclaimed as a breakthrough in health care, applied kinesiology is one of the most exciting developments in energetic medicine. It combines aspects of traditional Chinese medicine with a newly devised system of diagnosis and treatment. Instead of trying to identify or find the cause of a problem through symptoms, a practitioner tests specific muscles for strength or weakness. By its responses, the body itself apparently indicates the nature of any imbalances it may have, and the practitioner reads these responses to identify the best way of restoring health.

ORIGINS

The method was conceived in the United States during the 1960s by Dr. George Goodheart, a chiropractor who had a reputation for teaching innovative approaches. Goodheart realized that different parts of the body corresponded to those of established reflex points, as in the meridian system of traditional Chinese medicine. This was a major development for diagnosis of medical problems. It enabled a practitioner to "ask" the body questions by pressing reflex points, and the responses would indicate which areas were causing the problem. Kinesiology grew slowly at first, but once a solid base was established, interest turned into enthusiasm, and a bewildering number of specializations proliferated.

TRAINING

The training of practitioners in applied kinesiology is strict and uncompromising. The International College of Applied Kinesiology (ICAK) in Shawnee Mission, Kansas, was founded in the 1970s and reflects Dr. Goodheart's view that applied kinesiology should be kept in the hands of professionals. Entry onto the initial course is restricted to medical and other health professionals who have completed full-time four-year training—notably doctors, dentists, chiropractors, and osteopaths.

PHILOSOPHY AND METHOD

The basis of applied kinesiology is muscle testing. The patient, usually clothed, sits or lies down while the muscles on both sides of the body are tested. A muscle being tested is put under tension by the patient resisting the kinesiologist's opposing pressure, which is exaggerated for a few seconds. If the patient's resistance holds against this pressure, the muscle is deemed strong; if it gives way, it is deemed weak. The responses are then matched up with the bodily functions that relate to the particular muscle.

Each major muscle has several reflex points that relate to different functions of

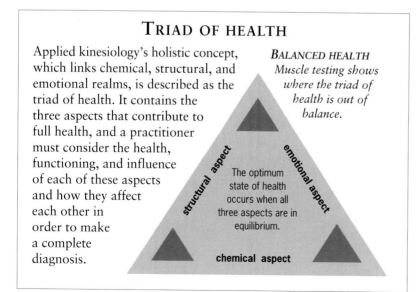

TRIAD OF HEALTH

Applied kinesiology's holistic concept, which links chemical, structural, and emotional realms, is described as the triad of health. It contains the three aspects that contribute to full health, and a practitioner must consider the health, functioning, and influence of each of these aspects and how they affect each other in order to make a complete diagnosis.

BALANCED HEALTH
Muscle testing shows where the triad of health is out of balance.

structural aspect
emotional aspect

The optimum state of health occurs when all three aspects are in equilibrium.

chemical aspect

TOUCH FOR HEALTH

Touch For Health is a simplification of the applied kinesiology technique, made accessible for nonhealth professionals and ordinary people to do at home. It is based on the same relationship of muscles to reflex points as in applied kinesiology and also relies on muscle testing, but involves fewer muscles than in the original method.

The system originated when Dr. Thie, a colleague of Goodheart's, set out guidelines in the very successful book

Touch For Health, published in 1973. The Touch For Health Foundation was then set up to train teachers, set educational standards, and continue research. Teaching emphasizes Touch For Health as a technique for the lay public, although many health professionals have also taken it up.

A system of self-enhancement rather than a professional qualification, it is often used by families of the chronically ill, so that relief is always at hand.

---

the body, and these are carefully mapped. This gives the kinesiologist a comprehensive reference that can be used to assess blood, lymph, and energy flow, nutritional and structural problems, and emotional imbalances. The applied kinesiologist knows how to ask questions and read the body's answers, building up a diagnostic statement.

The reflex points are themselves used to balance energies and relieve problems in combination with the acupressure points. Typically they are held tightly for half a minute until the pulses are felt to synchronize, often with accompanying sensations of moving energy.

Stress relief

Applied kinesiology also uses reflex points to treat emotional problems. It was discovered, after working with people in distress, that stimulation of two points on the forehead draws blood forward from the "reptilian brain" (an area connected to stress function) to the free-thinking frontal lobes. This allows better perspective. The external stress factors don't change but the patient's perception does.

Allergy testing

Testing for food allergies is a growing area in applied kinesiology research, although it is unknown whether successes are the result of methodology or pure intuition. Usually the suspected allergen is placed in the mouth but not swallowed. In some derivative techniques, however, many more substances are tested during a session by simply placing them one at a time in a glass phial on the abdomen. Allergic substances typically cause a weakening, usually in the muscles

that are related to digestion in the meridian system. A list is then compiled of foods to avoid, with a separate list of foods that are safe when eaten in moderation.

PROBLEMS TREATED

Practitioners say that applied kinesiology aims to restore whole-body balance, focusing on the underlying causative factors of an illness or condition. Most people would benefit from fine-tuning, especially when ill, and for this reason therapists feel they have something beneficial to offer most of the population. The system seems to be particularly helpful for relieving long-standing chronic conditions that have resolutely resisted regular approaches. An emphasis is also placed on its role in preventative health care; many future health problems manifest themselves as imbalances that are detectable by applied kinesiology.

CONTRAINDICATIONS

There are no contraindications to this therapy. The treatment essentially works with the body's own preferences and is simply aimed at increasing a patient's vital force and diagnosing potential problem areas. However, it is important to realize that applied kinesiology should not take the place of conventional medical treatment for long-term or serious conditions or illnesses. A practitioner can inform you if you should be getting help from other sources, including your primary-care doctor or a specialist.

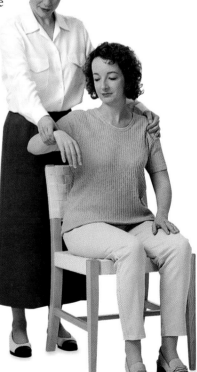

MUSCLE TESTING
A practitioner locates the source of the problem by feeling the patient's muscle responses to applied pressure.

EDUCATIONAL KINESIOLOGY

With special exercises and pressure on certain points to stimulate communication and thought processes, the brain can be trained to listen, understand, and learn more efficiently.

Touch therapies have long been used for physical and emotional problems. Educational kinesiology, a series of exercises, is now being used to enhance mental ability by improving the flow of information around the brain and encouraging better and quicker thinking.

ORIGINS

Educational kinesiology was developed in the 1970s by Dr. Paul Dennison, an educational therapist. He realized that kinesiology could be used to increase the brain's ability to learn by stimulating neuron pathways through the brain and thus enhancing natural mental abilities. The Brain Gym he devised is a series of simple exercises that teachers can use to help children concentrate for longer periods and learn more effectively.

TRAINING

In the United States training is overseen by the Educational Kinesiology Foundation, Ventura, California. In Canada training is coordinated by the Edu-K Brain Gym Learning Centre, Winnipeg, Manitoba.

PHILOSOPHY AND METHOD

Special exercises are used to stimulate the flow of information around the brain, with an emphasis on getting both sides of the brain to work in harmony. An inability to work to our potential is largely associated with stress, fatigue, and mental overload. Under stress, we often feel stuck because we are confined to one side of the brain—usually in a desperate attempt to simplify things so that we can sort them out quickly. This means that we are functioning in either the left side of the brain, which deals with logic, numbers, language, and comprehension, or the right side, the seat of emotions, intuition, and creativity, which help us to understand ideas. The goal is to move freely between one side and the other.

PROBLEMS TREATED

Educational kinesiology initially grew out of work designed to help people who have dyslexia and learning difficulties. It has now been developed into a system that can be useful for everyone. It can help improve mental functions such as concentration, reading, writing, and memory, and has also proved effective in stress control.

CONVENTIONAL OPINION

Educational kinesiology is acceptable to medical practitioners who can grasp the basic idea of improving cerebral coordination through a scientific system of therapy.

CLASSROOM HELP
Educational kinesiology is the application of pressure to specific points to enable students to listen, concentrate, and understand better.

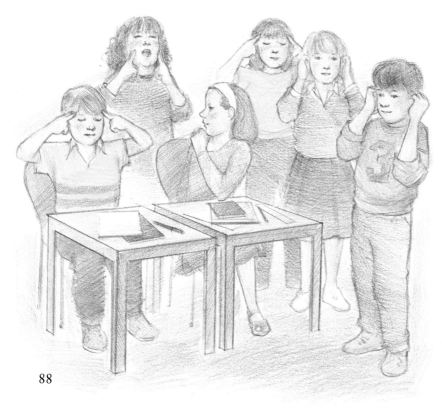

Improve Your Thinking with

Brain Gym Exercises

Stimulating nerve reaction and enhancing muscle use can help anyone see, hear, speak, and think more quickly and clearly. Doing these exercises for a few minutes before an important meeting or exam will enable you to focus your mental energies.

These exercises will stretch muscles in your face, head, shoulders, and neck, which are linked to nerves in your brain that control the internal connections of your brain, ears, and eyes. The exercises can also release any muscle tensions that develop from bad posture and provide stress relief, thus increasing your ability to tackle problems more easily.

> **BRAIN GYM**
>
> Courses about Brain Gym are given at numerous centers in the U.S. and Canada. Details about these, plus many books on the subject, are available from the organizations mentioned under "Training," opposite page.

POSITIVE POINTS

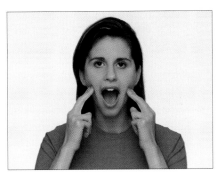

Lightly press two fingers on each side of your forehead, about halfway down, and hold for 3 to 10 minutes. This will relieve tension and increase blood flow to and around the brain.

THE ENERGY YAWN

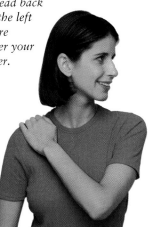

Open your mouth wide, as if to yawn, and massage the jaw muscles at the joints. It will relax your vision by stretching muscles between the jaw and skull, which also control the eye muscles.

THE THINKING CAP

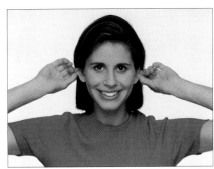

Pull the tops of your ears with your fingers, then move down your ear, pulling gently outward and pinching. When you reach the lobe, pull down. This stimulates hearing and sharpens comprehension.

THE OWL

1 *Squeeze the muscles of your right shoulder with your left hand, breathing in. Breathe out and turn your head slowly to the right until you are looking over your right shoulder.*

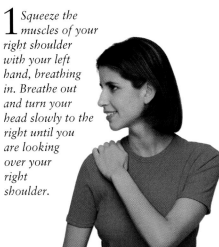

2 *Breathing in, turn your head back around to the left until you are looking over your left shoulder.*

3 *Breathing out, return your head to the center and rest your chin on your chest. Breathing deeply, let your head and shoulders relax. Repeat with the opposite side.*

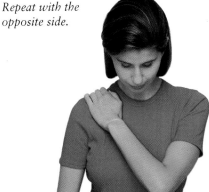

SHIATSU

Based on one of the oldest and most powerful forms of touch therapy, shiatsu takes its philosophy from the ancient Oriental concept of yin and yang, the contrasting forces of life.

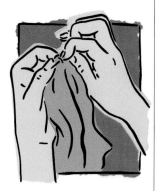

IMPROVING YOUR TOUCH

Both dressmaking and embroidery can improve the sensitivity of your fingertips. Running material through your hands, feeling its texture, its strength, the line of the weave, and the way it hangs, tells you how to work with it.

Shiatsu is a form of acupressure born out of traditional Oriental medicine. The name is Japanese for "finger pressure." Although fingers are the primary tools, all usable points of the therapist's body are sometimes called upon in treatment, including the thumbs, elbows, heels of the hands, forearms, and even knees, all applied in an economical way. The patient lies on a futon or mat on the floor, and the practitioner applies pressure to different parts of the body in order to balance the flow of life force energy, known in Japan as ki (qi in Chinese). The shiatsu practitioner is looking to restore a healthy integrity to the body's energy system.

ORIGINS

About the 10th century, traditional Chinese medicine found its way to Japan, most likely with Buddhist monks. The system taken there was Tao Yin, a combination of acupressure, massage, and breathing exercises representing the highest level of traditional Chinese medicine and focused on the harmonious flowing of subtle energies.

In the early 20th century, a book called *Shiatsu ho* by Tamai Tempaka reformulated the ancient art into a modern system that acknowledged Western anatomy and physiology, and a new era for shiatsu was born.

Shiatsu is now the most widely practiced of the acupressure systems in the West, and many different approaches exist. Most contain the same elements but emphasize certain ones over others. For example, some are concerned mainly with releasing blockages at the acupressure points. Others focus on more general body work and the balancing of the yin energy, which is quiet and deep, with the yang energy, which is active and on the surface. Still other approaches concentrate more on the interaction of the Five Elements (see opposite page).

PHILOSOPHY AND METHOD

To change the quality and quantity of ki, pressure is applied to specific points on the body surface called tsubo, which correspond to acupressure points in traditional Chinese medicine. The resulting changes affect the flow of vitalizing and organizing energy along energy pathways, or meridians. Shiatsu is concerned with an essential and subtle system that irrigates the body with vital energy, and practitioners believe that too much can be as bad as too little.

There are 12 major meridians, each supplying energy that is connected to the functioning of a specific organ or system in the body. Divided among these 12 meridians are some 700 tsubos through which the therapist can fine-tune a bodily system by either a stimulating or a calming pressure.

To bring about balance, accurate diagnosis is of paramount importance, and the principles of yin and yang and the Five Elements are applied to measure the balance of energy in the system. Diagnosis involves a search for characteristic signs and symptoms of yang/yin or elemental imbalance—for example, in the face or on the tongue—or for recognizable signs of trouble in specific meridians. Skills in observing, listening, questioning, and feeling the ki form the basis of good diagnosis, and they can take years to master fully. Once diagnosed, the

DID YOU KNOW?
The Yellow Emperor's Canon of Internal Medicine, written about 500 B.C., was a vast compilation of traditional remedies and philosophies, including the yin and yang principles. The Canon forms the basis for traditional Chinese medicine and most other Asian healing systems, including shiatsu, reflexology, polarity therapy, and Reiki.

THE FIVE ELEMENTS

The five elements of water, wood, fire, earth, and metal are all seen as aspects and manifestations of the one basic energy, or ki. These same elements are considered to be the building blocks of the whole universe, including our human bodies, and so provide a direct relationship between ourselves and our environment, its seasons, colors, and moods. Each element physically governs a meridian and organ function and is also characterized by an aspect of human emotion or personality. These are used to diagnose any imbalance in a person's ki. A problem would then be treated via the acupressure points.

FIVE ELEMENTS
During diagnosis, the therapist reads the relationships between the elements to help identify the patient's problem. For example, water controls fire, and if water is suppressed through illness, then fire will be unchecked, leading to overexcitement and nervousness.

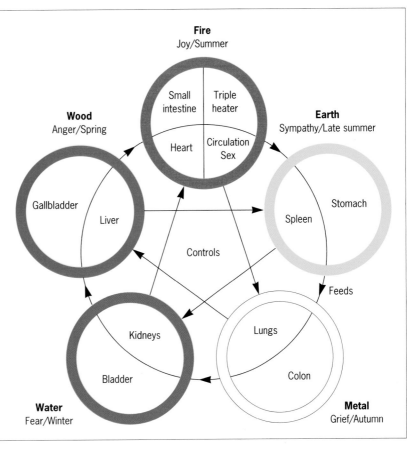

yang/yin imbalance is remedied by stimulating meridian points to balance energy flows.

TRAINING

Shiatsu schools have proliferated, and there is now a foundation of professional self-regulating bodies to oversee standards of education and ethics. In most courses in the United States, it takes three years of intense part-time study to achieve a professional level of competence. Training in Canada ranges from 300 to 2,200 hours, with most practitioners having 1,000 hours.

PROBLEMS TREATED

Strictly speaking, shiatsu has always been seen as a preventative approach to medicine; by treating the fundamental energy system of the body, it eliminates the causes of disease. The balancing of body energies improves many basic bodily functions and has a positive overall effect, improving digestion, vitality, and immune function, and detoxifying the system.

Today shiatsu is also used for healing, with concentration on causative factors rather than symptoms. Constipation and headaches respond well, as do bodily stiffness and muscular tensions generally. Shiatsu also has a great ability to relieve stress and calm the nervous system. Women with menstrual problems have found shiatsu helpful, and it can ease the discomforts and pain of pregnancy and childbirth.

CONTRAINDICATIONS

Shiatsu is contraindicated for anyone who has a high fever or possibly internal bleeding or a twisted gut. Sites of skin conditions, burns, bruises, and varicose veins should be avoided, although treatment can still be given. Pregnancy responds well to shiatsu, but a practitioner must avoid the lower legs, because pressure there could lead to miscarriage. Caution is also advised for people with fractures, skin infections, cancer, or disorders of the heart, liver, kidneys, or lungs.

CONVENTIONAL OPINION

As long as contraindications are considered, most doctors are happy for their patients to receive shiatsu in a preventive or stress-relieving capacity. There remains some skepticism about its usefulness for dealing with more serious conditions; medical care should be sought for any ongoing or major disorder.

FUNDAMENTALS OF JAPANESE HEALTH

The Japanese believe that health comes from your whole lifestyle, which is an integration of energies affected by everything that you do.

▶ *Diet should be well balanced and include a mixture of the five tastes—sweet, sour, hot, bitter, and salty.*

▶ *Stimulants and drugs should be avoided, including caffeine, alcohol, and nicotine.*

▶ *Exercise should be done regularly to raise the heartbeat and increase ki.*

▶ *The body should be protected from harsh external conditions, such as cold and dampness.*

Shiatsu Practitioner

Shiatsu is about balance and harmony, both within ourselves and between us and our environment. It can help offset the stresses and strains of success-based Western society, offering relaxation and peace of mind and rebalancing internal systems.

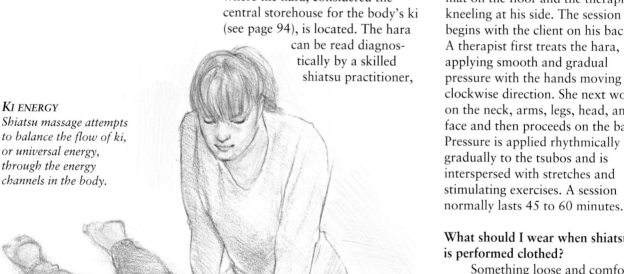

Bitter Grapefruit   **Sweet** Honey

Salty Rock salt   **Hot** Chilies   **Sour** Yogurt

A BALANCED DIET
According to shiatsu practice, a good diet consists of a balance of the five tastes— sweet, salty, bitter, sour, and hot. This enables an individual to achieve harmony and balance with the Five Elements.

KI ENERGY
Shiatsu massage attempts to balance the flow of ki, or universal energy, through the energy channels in the body.

What happens during a typical shiatsu session?

A session always starts with diagnosis, which will direct how the practitioner will proceed on this occasion; nothing is taken for granted. The diagnosis is made by questioning, observing, and touching. Particular attention is paid to the flow of ki in the meridians and also to the abdominal area, which is where the hara, considered the central storehouse for the body's ki (see page 94), is located. The hara can be read diagnostically by a skilled shiatsu practitioner, and the dynamic state of health of the whole body perceived.

Evaluating the yin and yang balance is also important. A patient who is fatigued, for example, would be diagnosed as being in a yin state. In this case, a shiatsu practitioner would try to stimulate yang energy.

Treatment takes place with the patient, usually clothed but sometimes unclothed, lying on a futon or mat on the floor and the therapist kneeling at his side. The session begins with the client on his back. A therapist first treats the hara, applying smooth and gradual pressure with the hands moving in a clockwise direction. She next works on the neck, arms, legs, head, and face and then proceeds on the back. Pressure is applied rhythmically and gradually to the tsubos and is interspersed with stretches and stimulating exercises. A session normally lasts 45 to 60 minutes.

What should I wear when shiatsu is performed clothed?

Something loose and comfortable is appropriate, preferably of cotton, as synthetics generate static electricity that can disturb ki. Sweatpants and a T-shirt are ideal.

What should I expect to feel after a shiatsu session?

Everyone reacts in an individual way, and this will change from treatment to treatment. However, it is not uncommon for an acutely ill or chronically unwell person to

MOXA AND CUPPING

Moxa and cupping are techniques commonly used by Shiatsu practitioners. Moxa is the application of heat to an acupressure point by burning a dried piece of the herb mugwort on top of a slice of ginger on the skin. Cupping is done by placing heated glass suction cups over an area to draw tissue into them and stimulate increased blood flow.

experience a "healing crisis." The person might feel stiff, tired, lethargic, or suffer headaches for one or two days. This is the body readjusting to a higher level of vitality and often means that toxins are being released. As health returns, these unpleasant reactions are usually replaced with feelings of lightness and vitality.

Can shiatsu be combined with Western medicine?

Although the two schools view patients very differently, they are both ultimately aiming to increase levels of health. Because they work on a patient on different levels, the combining of conventional medical care with shiatsu therapy has proved to be highly beneficial. More and more patients are finding that the deep relaxation induced by shiatsu seems to enhance healing without the risks associated with drugs.

Do you have to be ill to benefit?

The whole emphasis in shiatsu is on prevention rather than cure. In fact, in certain branches of the practice, this idea was taken to extremes at one point when practitioners refused to treat people who were ill. They did not want to waste their energy on anyone who had ignorantly not practiced proper prevention and taken shiatsu regularly.

Are there advantages to an Oriental diagnosis over a conventional one?

A shiatsu diagnosis really comes into its own in cases of chronic ill health. Western medicine's approach to most situations is practiced, well defined, and normally well applied, but there are weaknesses in bringing relief from chronic conditions. Very often chronic conditions are the result of ongoing stresses, and it is here that the Oriental approach excels. Its success is based on its truly holistic vision, taking into account energy-balancing, emotional and psychological factors and our relationship with the elements and the environment around us.

How many treatments are needed?

Just as some conditions have taken time to arise, realistically they will take time to reverse. Typically, many will need five to seven treatments, normally on a weekly basis, and then an evaluation can be made as to whether more treatment is needed. However, shiatsu's primary concern is preventing illness and establishing and maintaining a good level of health. Many people go for treatment once every month or so to help achieve this state.

Is shiatsu safe during pregnancy?

Shiatsu can be beneficial to women during pregnancy and childbirth and is believed even to aid conception in some cases. However, care needs to be taken during the first three months. After this period, the mother can be helped into a balanced state, which also eases backache and pain during childbirth.

AFTER TOUCH THERAPY

A good way to complement your shiatsu treatment is with Do-in, a series of exercises based on shiatsu. It is designed to stimulate the meridian system through breathing, stretching, and meditation. When energy meridians are stretched, this permits the even flow of energy.

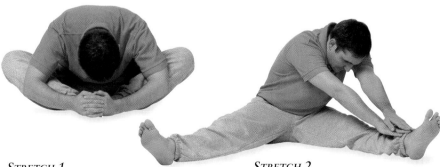

STRETCH 3
Standing with your toes touching a wall, raise your left arm and place your palm against the wall. Take your right foot in your right hand and press your thigh firmly against the wall. Bend your head backward and hold for 10 seconds, stretching the front of your body. Repeat on the other side.

STRETCH 1
Sit with your legs open and the soles of your feet touching. Put your hands around your feet and bend slowly forward, bringing your forehead down toward your toes.

STRETCH 2
Sit up straight with your legs extended and as far apart as possible. Slide your hands slowly down your left leg. Repeat with the other leg.

JIN SHIN

The ancient Japanese art of Jin Shin involves the treatment of energy centers within the body. A session releases stress, promotes relaxation, and rebalances and revitalizes the system.

The Jin Shin energy system can be likened to a circuit cable that carries universal energy throughout the body. Energy locks or centers occur in specific places on the cable, and when these become blocked by stress and toxins, health problems result. Jin Shin clears the locks to allow the free passage of energy, thus revitalizing the body and restoring health to it.

The therapy has become popular in recent years for relieving tension and treating stress-related disorders such as myalgic encephalomyelitis, more commonly known as chronic fatigue syndrome, and also for treating depression and digestive disorders.

ORIGINS

Although it is not clear how or when Jin Shin originated, it is thought that it emerged before or alongside the traditional Chinese system of meridians and acupressure points. The Jin Shin system more or less disappeared for centuries until it was revitalized by Jiro Murai in Japan in the 1960s. American practitioners, introduced to the therapy by Mary Burmeister, adopted Jin Shin. Since then it has undergone further developments, and related practices have emerged, including Jin Shin Ki, Jin Shin Do, and Jin Shin Jyutsu, all of which have varied approaches to the subject.

Jin Shin Do was founded in California in the late 1960s by Iona Marsaa Teeguarden, who drew together elements of several systems to promote happiness and contentment. The emphasis of Jin Shin Do is on the reconnection with the emotional and higher self through deep relaxation and careful rebalancing of the energy system.

Roselyn Journeaux was the first British practitioner of the art of Jin Shin and the founder of Jin Shin Ki (see opposite page).

TRAINING

Because Jin Shin practitioners are not regulated by any governing body, you must do your own checking to determine that your trainer or practitioner is adequately qualified. Length of training and practice give some indication of a practitioner's level of experience and expertise, but the best way to find a good one is by recommendation.

There are official training courses in the United States that cover Jin Shin and the related schools, including Jin Shin Jyutsu, Inc., in Arizona, the Jin Shin Do Foundation in California, and High Touch in Washington State. Also, practitioners who have studied with Mary Burmeister or one of her students are usually well qualified. In Canada a qualified practitioner will have studied at the Canadian Acupressure Institute of Victoria, B.C., which offers a 725-hour training program in Jin Shin Do,

HARA BREATHING

Healing energy is believed to come from the hara, a reservoir of energy in the abdomen about two finger widths below the navel. It can be replenished using special breathing techniques. Place your hands over your hara. As you breathe in, count to five and imagine the breath going straight into your abdomen. Visualize a golden stream of water pouring into a pool or fuel stoking a large fire. Hold your breath for the count of five, exhale, and relax, keeping your focus on the hara. Repeat until breathing becomes a seamless cycle of inhaling, holding, and exhaling.

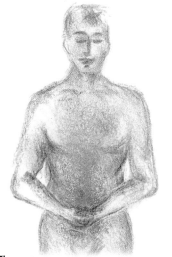

THE HARA
The hara is located in the abdomen a couple of inches below the navel, although it can encompass the whole pelvic area.

JIN SHIN KI

Developed by Roselyn Journeaux during the mid-1990s, Jin Shin Ki forms part of a comprehensive therapy that includes flower remedies, Chinese food herbs, lymphatic drainage massage (see page 42), and healing and diagnostic elements of various Asian and Oriental therapies.

Journeaux used her own knowledge and experience of healing and diagnosis, as well as the established systems, to develop ASHM—the Association of Self-Help Medicine. This uses a unique diagnostic system in which a patient is asked about his or her past. Be prepared to answer questions about when you had illnesses, injuries, or major changes in your life and about your family history and intimate relationships. The answers are thought to indicate any weaknesses or imbalances in your system. The diagnosis relates different illnesses and diseases to personality and lifestyle disorders and gives indications to deeper unresolved problems.

Other diagnostic techniques are brought in, including tongue, teeth, and hair analyses of Ayurveda (see page 50); the Five Elements system (see page 91); and age and astrology analyses.

Once the diagnosis has been worked out, the therapist will decide which parts of the body need attention and will hold the energy centers, in pairs, until a pulse of energy is felt. Self-help exercises are emphasized, and you will be given a series of exercises to do at home.

Self-help exercises

This basic stress reliever, which can be done anywhere, will help you balance your energy. The pulse is the contraction of the blood vessel, felt as a subtle, rhythmic vibration, that pulsates throughout the whole finger.

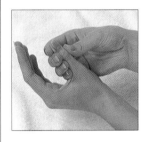

HOLD THE PULSE
Press your left thumb between the fingers and thumb of your right hand and feel for the pulse.

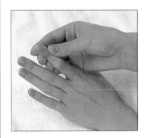

REPEAT ON ALL FINGERS
In the same way, squeeze your left index finger until you feel a steady, rhythmic pulse. Continue to do the same with all the fingers on your left hand and then the thumb and fingers of your right hand.

or at one of the American institutions mentioned previously. If you plan to take a Jin Shin course yourself, find out as much as possible about available courses and the level of qualification that each will give you.

PHILOSOPHY AND METHOD

Jin Shin is based on the idea that on each side of the body there are 26 locks, or energy centers, that regulate the body's energy system. The locks become closed when a body is stressed, filled with toxins, or out of balance with any aspect of its life or environment. Jin Shin practitioners reopen the locks by placing their hands over the energy centers in a specific sequence, based on a diagnosis. They can spend several minutes or longer on each pair of locks. Practitioners often say that there may even be a slight swelling if a lock is heavily congested, and a tingling sensation can be felt as a center is unblocked. During each session the patient is clothed—a loose, cotton sweat suit is ideal—and jewelry and shoes are removed.

Both the physical and emotional health of a patient is considered within a Taoist context: the achievement of balance through an understanding of and feeling for harmony with the energies of the universe.

PROBLEMS TREATED

Jin Shin can be applied to a wide range of problems, but because it aims to return the whole body to balance and high vitality, it can be particularly helpful in enhancing all-round health, including circulation, hair condition, complexion, the immune system, and emotional and spiritual balance. Basically, Jin Shin brings harmony and regularity to the functions of your whole being.

It has been found to be especially beneficial for sufferers of chronic fatigue syndrome, depression, asthma, and digestive disorders. Treatments have also been known to help in cases of cancer, leukemia, and autism.

CONTRAINDICATIONS

There are no contraindications to Jin Shin, especially since there is no pressure on the body. It involves no rubbing or massage. Everyone can benefit from the relaxation and fine-tuning of the treatment, and it can be used at home for self-help treatment.

CONVENTIONAL OPINION

Like most energy rebalancing therapies, Jin Shin is becoming more well known and now meets with less skepticism than when it first arrived in the West. The concept that illnesses and diseases are caused by emotional problems is more widely accepted than in years past. Most doctors would not object to Jin Shin as a general health tool, although it would not be appropriate to use it for specific health problems. You should consult your general practitioner if you have a serious or chronic condition.

REIKI

Reiki has spread quickly as a way of restoring natural energy and health. Based on Eastern philosophies, it has captured the imagination and enthusiasm of millions worldwide.

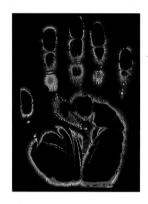

ELECTROPHOTOGRAPHY
Also known as Kirlian photography, electrophotography shows energy emanating from the body and forming an aura.

REIKI TREATMENT
The hands of a practitioner are placed on the body of a patient, allowing the passage of energy from one to the other. Sometimes the hands are simply placed within a person's aura rather than actually touching the body, to the same effect.

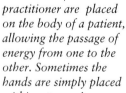

In Reiki (pronounced ray-kee), healing is carried out through the transference of energy from the healer to the patient. It is based on the principle that universal energy is present in everyone, and so it is not exclusive and does not depend on any belief system. Part of the appeal of Reiki lies in its simplicity. It has been presented as a tool for personal and global transformation.

ORIGINS

Reiki was rediscovered in the 19th century by a Japanese Buddhist monk, Dr. Mikao Usui, who embarked on a search to find the secret of spiritual healing—a search that took him 14 years. He was meditating on a mountain when, at the darkest point of the night, he saw a piercing light approaching him. He believed that it contained the answer to the secret of spiritual healing and also that if the light struck him it might kill him. He decided in that moment that learning how to heal others was of more value than his own life, so he allowed himself to be struck and fell into a deep trance. It was then revealed to him that the key to healing was to be found in Sanskrit symbols in the Sutras, the Buddhist scriptures. Dr. Usui had experienced the first Reiki attunement, and he realized that he had rediscovered an ancient art of spiritual healing.

Reiki is learned by attunement, or initiation, from a Reiki master, a system that reflects its Oriental origins. Dr. Usui initiated 16 Reiki masters before his death in 1926, and various groups have descended from the different masters. Mrs. Hawayo Takata, a Hawaiian master, has probably been the most influential in the spread of Reiki throughout North America and Europe. Since Takata's death in 1980, several branches of Reiki have evolved, many claiming to be the only authentic therapy. The differences lie mainly in the addition of other healing techniques, the methods of teaching initiates, and the number of levels of attainment.

There is something divine about Reiki healing, yet paradoxically the organizations that have sprung up around it are very human. Mrs. Takata devised a high fee structure in order to command respect for the therapy. This has led to an increasing number of independent, nontraditional teachers who do not belong to any of the official organizations and who offer Reiki at lower prices to make it more accessible. This situation has inevitably caused confusion concerning the integrity of the healing philosophy and the validity of different groups.

TRAINING

Generally there are three levels of attainment—Reiki I, II, and III—with each one increasing the positive power of the energy, or ki, and allowing new practitioners to treat others and themselves and perform absent healing. Training has now become less exclusive, although courses can still be difficult to find outside the United States.

THE SPIRITUAL NATURE OF REIKI

Reiki is regarded as sacred, but it is not a religion and asks for no special faith or beliefs other than faith in the ability to heal through Reiki energy. This energy is seen as coming from a universal force or spirit, and the practice of Reiki is essentially spiritual in nature. It can be thought of as the giving of the energy received during meditation—a sharing of it rather than a focusing on it.

PHILOSOPHY AND METHOD

The name Reiki derives from two Japanese words: *rei,* meaning universal spiritual consciousness, and *ki,* meaning universal life force. The healing is achieved by giving ki to the person being treated. In order to do this, a practitioner must be in tune with the universal spiritual consciousness, and his or her own life force channels must be open so that ki flows freely through them. Learning the art of Reiki therefore demands spiritual attunement, or initiation, which makes Reiki practitioners significantly different from most other healers, although established healers often report increased healing power after receiving Reiki attunements.

The universal energy heals by restoring diminished areas of energy flow in a patient. Poor energy flow or blocked energy is brought about by toxicity or structural faults in the body, inadequate exercise, poor nutrition, or negative thoughts, and opens the door to illness—physical and/or mental. Practitioners lay their hands over areas of diminished energy in patients and recharge them with positive energy, thus restoring the life force and with it a person's health and vitality.

PROBLEMS TREATED

Reiki, like other energy rebalancing therapies, views illness as a disruption of the body's energy systems. It aims to restore fundamental energy circulation and thus improve general health and well-being. The emphasis is more on cause than symptoms and can be beneficial for patients of all kinds. Reiki can work alongside conventional health measures, often improving results and minimizing pain and stress.

CONTRAINDICATIONS

Reiki does not address specific illnesses or conditions—it treats the person, not the disease—and it does not involve any physical pressure or manipulation. Because of this approach, there are no contraindications.

CONVENTIONAL OPINION

The main concern would be the possible dangers of extravagant claims and missed diagnoses if treatment prevents a patient from seeking medical supervision. However, the obvious benefits of a relaxing healing session are recognized by most doctors, and it is generally promoted in this respect. There is much evidence that Reiki can play an important, positive, and comforting role in easing the pain of long-term illnesses.

THE FIVE STAGES TO ENLIGHTENMENT

Reiki enhances the process of healing and progression on the Path to Enlightenment. The aim is to release oneself from earthly attachments and gain freedom from pain by stepping out of the body and concentrating on the spirit. The five stages on the Path to Enlightenment are listed below.

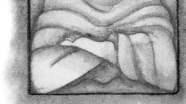

Stage 5: Enlightenment
Element: Void or Spirit
Process: The Ninth
  Consciousness
Color: Blue

Stage 4: Spiritual body
Element: Wind
Process: The Five Senses
Color: Black

Stage 3: Mental body
Element: Fire
Process: The Mind
Color: Red

Stage 2: Emotional body
Element: Water
Process: The Passions
Color: White

Stage 1: Physical body
Element: Earth
Process: The Consciousness
Color: Yellow

*THE PATH TO ENLIGHTENMENT
Each of the five stages is represented by a body part, an element, a color, and a Reiki symbol for the spiritual level.*

The Reiki Healer

Channeling universal energy through the Reiki healer into the subject's body demands the clearing of the healer's energy channels and a full understanding of the nature of spiritual energy and the personal energies of the subject and the healer.

REIKI IDEALS

Dr. Usui advised that the following mantra be repeated every day so that patients could actively meet Reiki halfway and not remain merely passive recipients of the therapy.

▶ *Just for today, I will let go of anger.*

▶ *Just for today, I will let go of worry.*

▶ *Just for today, I will give thanks for my blessings.*

▶ *Just for today, I will do my work honestly.*

▶ *Just for today, I will be kind to my neighbor and every living thing.*

How does Reiki energy heal?

A person is healthy when life energy, which vitalizes all bodily processes, is flowing freely and naturally within the body and in the external aura. This life force nourishes and supports, and when it is blocked or diminished, the body becomes open to depression or physical illness. Reiki heals by overcoming negative blocks with a surge of positive energy, enhancing self-image and bringing relief from problems concerned with negativity and depression.

What conditions can Reiki treat?

Reiki works in terms of giving healing to the whole person. The Reiki energy has an innate intelligence that directs it to where an individual needs it most. All health and emotional conditions will therefore benefit, often because the underlying energetic and emotional patterns are helped by the healing energy. There are many stories of miraculous healings connected to the application of Reiki, although it would be imprudent to have unrealistic expectations about what treatment can achieve.

With serious illness, Reiki healing should be performed as part of an overall approach that includes conventional allopathic medical supervision. Indeed, Reiki will often work favorably alongside a wide range of other treatments.

Who is able to learn Reiki?

Anyone with a desire to heal can learn Reiki. It is not necessary to have already demonstrated natural healing abilities or to possess any spiritual feelings. You are shown how to use your own healing powers, simply allowing energy to flow with the intention of healing. It doesn't even have to be practiced; the ability is retained for life.

What is a Reiki master?

A Reiki master is a person who is empowered to empower, someone who is authorized to initiate others into Reiki. This role requires a firm commitment to the purpose and

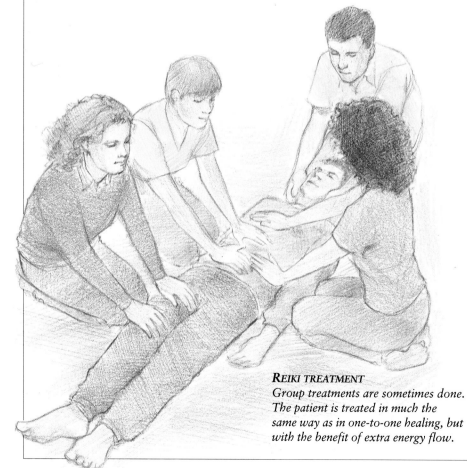

REIKI TREATMENT
Group treatments are sometimes done. The patient is treated in much the same way as in one-to-one healing, but with the benefit of extra energy flow.

spread of Reiki, and is filled by someone who has worked with the first- and second-degree stages and progressed to the third, master level. It is from a Reiki master that a new student receives the attunements, in which a special lifelong link to the Reiki source is created. It has been suggested that it is not the individual who masters Reiki, but the quiet spiritual energy of Reiki that masters the individual.

What happens during an attunement?

An attunement is a ceremony through which a Reiki student is given energy and special healing powers from a Reiki master. During the ceremony the student sits in a straight-backed chair with hands held palms together at chest height and feet flat on the floor. This allows the Reiki master to move around the student. Attunements may be done singly or, more often, in groups.

The heart of the initiation is the tracing of the Tibetan symbols over the hands, spine, and head of the student, accompanied by ceremonial tapping and blowing. The initiation constitutes a gentle ritual that perhaps reflects Reiki's Eastern origins, and the atmosphere generated is both respectful and sacred. It may be a simple process, but many people find this a powerful spiritual experience, reporting healings, visions, past life

experiences, and an increase in intuition. To prepare for the attunement, a student must have exercised the channeling of universal energy and studied the philosophy of Reiki. Reiki II and Master levels require further experience and a deeper knowledge and understanding of Reiki healing.

What are the ceremonial symbols?

The symbols used are a closely kept secret, not even revealed to students at Reiki I and disclosed only at levels II and III. The symbols represent and personify the sacred energies used in Reiki and embody this energy. To work for healing purposes, the symbols need to be drawn or visualized correctly, rather like using a key to open a door.

Has Reiki changed over the years?

The Reiki energy has not changed, but the teaching and organizations around it have. From modest beginnings, Reiki became an expensive and almost exclusively Western luxury. However, there has been a noticeable trend away from this in recent years, due to an influx of independent teachers who have challenged the official organizations. They are committed to the use of Reiki as a tool for global change and have made Reiki more accessible by reducing the fees.

Has any research been done on the health benefits of Reiki?

A five-year trial on the effects of Reiki used alongside conventional treatment has been started at Stanford University in the United States. Regular Reiki therapy has been given to 300 cancer patients who were diagnosed as terminally ill with only three months to live. After two and half years, over half the group is still alive and their quality of life has much improved. Those patients who died did so more comfortably than would have been anticipated. Much more research is now being carried out, especially on patients suffering from HIV-related illnesses and conditions that have stressful or painful side effects.

AFTER TOUCH THERAPY: YOGA

After a session with a Reiki healer, it is good to relax quietly by yourself for a while and enjoy the afterglow. The yoga positions below are ideal. Aim to hold each pose for at least 5 minutes and try to meditate as you

do so, concentrating on your body. Start with the tip of your toes and work up to the crown of your head, breathing deeply and feeling the basic pleasure of simply being alive.

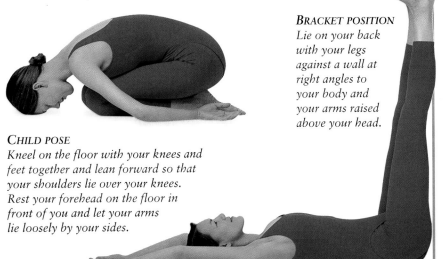

BRACKET POSITION
Lie on your back with your legs against a wall at right angles to your body and your arms raised above your head.

CHILD POSE
Kneel on the floor with your knees and feet together and lean forward so that your shoulders lie over your knees. Rest your forehead on the floor in front of you and let your arms lie loosely by your sides.

POLARITY THERAPY

Polarity therapy attempts to balance the positive and negative forces of the whole body using part of the Indian chakra system. It encompasses massage, diet, exercise, and counseling.

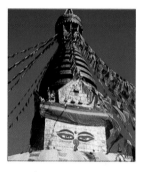

THE THIRD EYE
Many Eastern cultures represent universal energy being channeled to people through a third eye on the forehead.

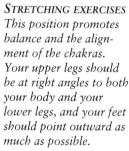

STRETCHING EXERCISES
This position promotes balance and the alignment of the chakras. Your upper legs should be at right angles to both your body and your lower legs, and your feet should point outward as much as possible.

Like many other energy rebalancing approaches, polarity therapy asserts that most illnesses develop because of blockages to the free flow of energy currents. Several techniques are used that combine both Western and Eastern approaches. The therapy attempts to remove blockages to energy, creating a state of neutral balance to allow full spiritual health.

ORIGINS

Polarity therapy was created in the middle of the 20th century by Dr. Randolph Stone, an Austrian living in the United States. It grew out of his disenchantment with the limitations of his work as a natural health practitioner. He kept seeing the same patients with the same recurring problems, and it seemed that there was an underlying pattern of illness constantly reasserting itself in each patient—often an age-old problem that had not been resolved. This prompted him to study more deeply, and he began to embrace Eastern energy-based philosophies.

Dr. Stone traveled widely in the East, particularly in India, where he was influenced by the chakra system, and his ideas began to take shape, although the whole method took more than 50 years to evolve fully. This was pioneering work, as awareness of auras and energy flow were far from commonplace in the West at the time, and many health care practitioners considered his ideas backward and lacking in plausibility. It was not until the 1960s that Dr. Stone's work became more accepted as people opened their minds to more spiritual healing concepts.

TRAINING

There are still few places outside the United States where practitioners are trained, but those available usually give a comprehensive course and award a proper certificate. Practitioners often come to polarity therapy from other alternative practices and bring methods from them into their practices.

PHILOSOPHY AND METHOD

Polarity therapy is based on the theory that to be truly healthy there has to be free circulation of the body's normal and natural energy currents and that illness represents a blockage in this process. Drawing largely from Ayurveda, yoga, and acupuncture, Dr. Stone came to see the body as a living magnet with a natural circulation of electromagnetic currents from positive to negative poles. His polarity therapy aims to restore normal circulation of currents where they have become disturbed or blocked. This is believed to banish the underlying cause of illness and thus prevent its recurrence.

Disturbances were seen to occur as a result of four main types of disorder: structural misalignments, physical toxicity, psy-

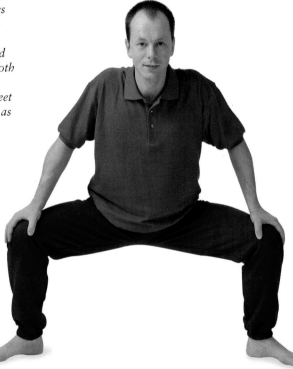

chological problems, and the effects of stress. Polarity therapy incorporates four natural ways of balancing energy, each one particularly appropriate to one of the four causes of disturbance: touching and manipulation, diet and detoxification, stretching and exercise, and counseling to change thoughts, lifestyle patterns, and attitudes.

This four-step approach is used to reorganize the energy flows of a patient into a healthy pattern based on the Indian concept of chakras, each symbolizing an element, a body part, a function, and an inner state. When the chakras are out of balance, the body does not function properly; if the imbalance is not redressed, a downward spiral of health problems can result. (Indian Ayurvedic medicine, from which Dr. Stone drew inspiration, recognizes seven chakras, but he chose just five, which correspond to the elements ether, air, fire, water, and earth.)

For example, a polarity therapist would see a man who has difficulty grounding himself in the world as having a water energy imbalance, or a woman who always fails to finish projects as needing her earth energy center rebalanced. The polarity therapist builds this picture from information based on a full case history combined with an analysis of energy pathways, reflexes, and posture. From the diagnosis a treatment is selected from Dr. Stone's four paths to health. Usually a combination of all four methods is used.

Manipulation and touch

Hands are used to balance the energy currents and five elements and disperse blockages by setting up a polarizing field between

THE CHAKRAS

Chakra is a Sanskrit word meaning wheel, and the chakras spin slowly or quickly depending on the energy passing through them. Chakras link the physical being with subtle energy, each one representing a function and an inner state. At the top of the body is the throat chakra, dealing with self-expression. Next is the heart chakra, concerned with self-love, then the central solar plexus chakra, which deals with self-worth. Below this comes the sacral chakra, then the base chakra, concerned with self-respect and self-awareness, respectively.

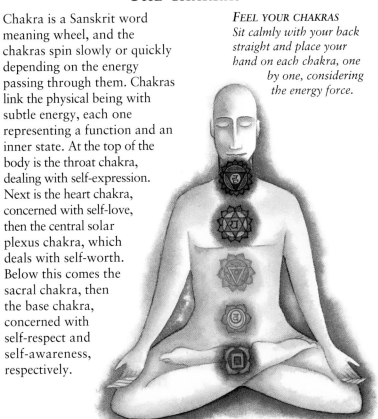

FEEL YOUR CHAKRAS
Sit calmly with your back straight and place your hand on each chakra, one by one, considering the energy force.

the two opposing forces. Three types of pressure are utilized: neutral, positive, and negative. Neutral consists of a soft, light touch with the fingertips to soothe and balance in a pleasing way. Positive pressure is the manipulation of various body parts to create movement. Negative pressure is deep and sometimes painful pressure and manipulations into the tissues to disperse stress

THE THREE CURRENTS

The chakras are formed from the three currents of universal energy, which enter the body through the third eye in the middle of the forehead. The currents spiral down the spine, and a chakra is formed at the place where the three currents cross over each other.

▶ *The* pingala *is the positively charged current.*

▶ *The* ida *is the negatively charged current.*

▶ *The* sushumna *is the neutral current.*

READING THE CHAKRAS

Diagnosis is carried out by considering a patient's physical, psychological, and emotional state in relation to the different chakra characteristics. For example, tonsillitis signifies a disorder in the throat chakra, indicating repressed expression.

CHAKRA	ELEMENT	BODY PART	FUNCTION	INNER STATE
Throat	Ether (space)	Throat, shoulders	Creativity	Intuition, synthesis
Heart	Air	Heart, lungs	Love	Compassion, love
Solar plexus	Fire	Digestive system	Will, drive	Intense emotion
Sacral	Water	Reproductive system	Pleasure, sexuality	Self-confidence
Base	Earth	Legs, feet, large intestine	Solidity, survival	Stability

and remove blockages. This leaves patients feeling relaxed, calm, and free of tension, ready for the three other elements that make up the whole of polarity therapy.

Stretching postures

Stretches are used primarily to remove energy blocks, although they will also strengthen and stretch muscles, ligaments, and the spine. They are based on stretching out the meridians and chakras to ease the flow of energy and relax tensions in the body. The patient is expected to let out sighs, shouts, and groans, releasing energies from within and adding a new dimension to the exercises. These are done mindfully, being careful not to overstrain and noting the physical, emotional, and mental reactions. The patient is often given a list of exercises to practice a few times a week at home.

Diet and detoxification

This phase starts with a two-week cleansing diet consisting of fresh fruits and vegetables and an increased fluid intake to expel accumulated clogging toxins. To help the liver detoxify, the one-day liver flush is given; it consists of a small cupful of olive oil, lemon juice, gingerroot, and garlic, taken four times throughout the day. A health-building diet follows for an extended period, and finally a maintenance diet, based on pure foods and vegetarian principles, is begun.

Counseling

Our lives and health are largely governed by attitudes born out of conditioning. In fact, many attitudes have been unconsciously conditioned in us from a young age by our parents, teachers, peers, and an increasingly important element, the media. Not all of these attitudes are life-enhancing. Counseling encourages patients to examine their long-held negative thoughts and beliefs and helps change these into more positive expressions of the spirit. It is important to feel relaxed during the sessions, because the therapist will try to locate what your spirit and your personality need and to identify any contradictions between them.

PROBLEMS TREATED

Polarity therapy is particularly good for anyone who is suffering from stress or has a stress-related illness, such as chronic fatigue syndrome. It can also relieve stomach problems, migraines, and allergies. Counseling can be useful for people who need to discuss or express their personal problems or who have tensions related to emotional stress.

CONTRAINDICATIONS

The manipulations can be deep and sometimes painful, and if you have any medical conditions or sore areas, you should inform the practitioner before treatment. The diets are not recommended for people who are weak or have eating disorders.

CONVENTIONAL OPINION

Many general practitioners are perplexed by the theory, but most would not quarrel with polarity therapy when it encourages their patients to take responsibility for their own health through massage, exercise, and counseling. However, doctors would probably have reservations about detoxifying diets.

THE AURA

Polarity therapy teaches that the body is surrounded by bands of energy that together form a person's aura. Each layer reflects an aspect of being: the aura is often known as the mirror of being. When a part of the being is repressed or overactive, illness or injury will result. Believers in the chakra system view every sign of ill health as an indication of chakra misalignment or repression of emotions and functions that relate to one of the chakras and need to be redressed.

SEEING AURAS
Clarity and definition of an aura can be seen by some clairvoyants, although it is thought to be felt by many people subconsciously.

The mental body develops with mental awareness, especially on a more abstract level, through meditation and deep understanding. People who have a highly developed mental field are thought to more readily receive intuitive ideas and thoughts, including clairvoyance and telepathy.

The etheric body, also known as the health aura or vital body, is the direct emanation of energy that surrounds the physical body. It is highly sensitive to thought processes and spirituality.

The astral body, also called the field of emotions or desire, reflects moods and feelings like sadness, love, anger, and anxiety. This body is more obvious and closer to the aura surface in people who have a less well developed mental field—for example, children.

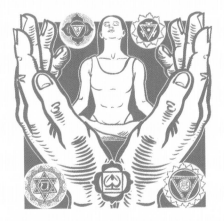

CHAPTER 5

MASSAGE REMEDIES

Whether you are suffering from a physical or an emotional complaint or just want to relieve tired muscles, massage can help. This chapter illustrates massage techniques for relaxation, recuperation, and relief from a range of conditions and problems. To boost health and refresh the spirit, follow the step-by-step sequences.

Lower Back Pain

Lower back pain can occur suddenly, debilitating the sufferer and disrupting lives. Back pain is often closely linked to emotional problems, and those going through a stressful period may find themselves with back pain for no apparent physical reason. A lower back massage can relieve muscle tension, although more crucially, it can relax and revitalize the recipient.

Massage can help relieve back pain that is associated with muscle disorders, but spine dysfunctions must be treated by an osteopath or orthopedic specialist. For muscular disorders the massage itself will depend on the exact problem. Listen to the recipient and find out where the pain is and what strokes or techniques are most effective at easing the pain or stretching out the painful muscles. Stroking and kneading are the best techniques to use; avoid pummeling and hacking, as they can damage the spine.

1 *Stroke the back from the base up the spine to the shoulders, then down the sides to the buttocks. Repeat several times. These movements have a highly soothing effect, releasing a great deal of tension and allowing the recipient to breathe more easily. After a few long strokes, ask where the problem areas are.*

LIFESTYLE TIPS

▶ Exercises are excellent for back problems. Try stretching the spine gently by leaning forward and backward every hour or so. Swimming exercises are particularly good for the back because the water supports the body and allows the muscles to be stretched without putting pressure on the spine (see pages 72–73).

▶ Try to make your life as stress-free as possible. Your bad back could be telling you that you need to slow down.

▶ Do not lie down or sit for long periods of time without a good stretch. If you work behind a desk, make sure that you get up and walk around or stretch every half hour or so.

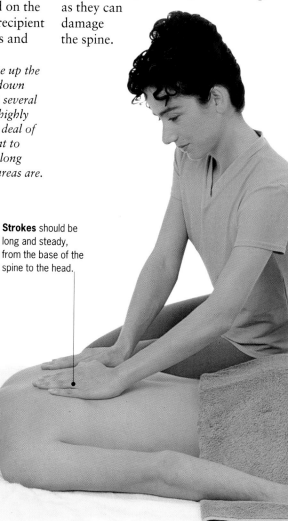

The recipient's head should face to one side, but keep the neck as straight as possible.

Strokes should be long and steady, from the base of the spine to the head.

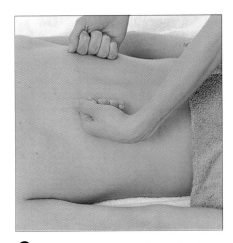

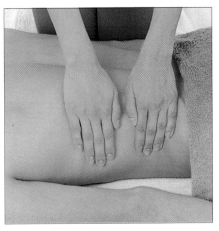

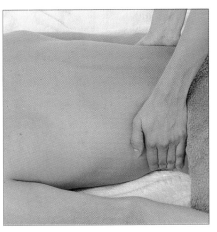

2 Cover the area of the lower back with a kneading movement to disperse muscle tension. Start gently and gradually knead more firmly. Take care when working on a particular problem area or on painful muscles.

3 Place your hands next to each other in the center of the back and stroke them firmly down the opposite side of the body. Bring them back to the central position. Repeat several times and then use the same action on the other side.

4 Place your hands on either side of the body and pull upward toward the spine alternately with one hand and then the other. Repeat six times and then reverse the process, starting at the spine and taking each hand down the side.

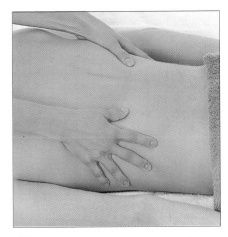

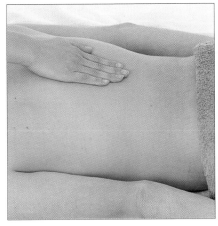

5 Kneeling at the recipient's head, start with your hands at the sides of the waist, then draw them up the back to the armpits, stretching the back with the palms of your hands.

6 Gently stroke down the lower back toward the buttocks, first with one hand and then with the other. This soothing action is deeply relaxing and conducive to talking over any problems.

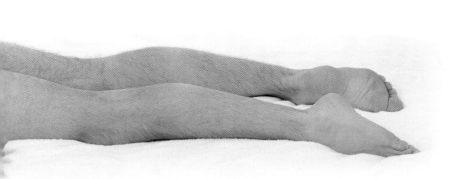

STRESS-RELATED BACK PROBLEMS

A lot of back pain is caused by worries and tensions building up in the muscles of the back. This is why so many people suffer from back problems when they are going through stressful events such as a breakdown in a marriage or a major problem at work. It is important to recognize where your stress is originating and try to understand and resolve it.

Often touch therapies bring to the fore a recognition that there are deeper issues to resolve. For example, if you realize that too many demands are being placed on you, you might consider taking a course in assertiveness to help you cope.

Alternatively, relaxation techniques and exercises can help reduce the effects of stress. In addition to a relaxing touch therapy, try meditation (see page 53) or taking a walk (see page 65).

Foot Cramp

Most people experience foot cramp from time to time, and it can be very painful and difficult to relieve. A cramp is a prolonged and painful spasm caused by the continual use of a muscle that is not given the chance to relax. It usually occurs in the limbs, especially in the feet, although it can also occur in the intestine or stomach, especially if you exercise immediately after eating.

A soothing massage for a foot cramp helps in a couple of different ways. First, it can ease a cramped muscle back to a relaxed position, forcing the contraction to stop. Second, it can improve circulation by stimulating the flow of fresh blood to the site and improving the distribution of oxygen to the muscles, thus inducing relaxation and reducing the spasm. Make sure that the cramped muscle is completely rested afterward to maintain circulation and prevent the muscle seizure from recurring.

1 *It is not necessary to undress for this massage, but the recipient should lie on his or her back and remove shoes and socks. Take the foot that is in spasm first and apply firm, soothing strokes over the entire foot. Encourage the recipient to relax; the muscle spasm will diminish greatly if breathing, and thus the supply of oxygen to the site, is normal.*

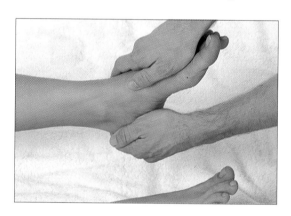

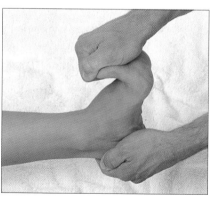

2 *If the pain continues to be acute, support the foot with one hand and stretch the foot and toes with the other. You may need to continue this action until the pain wears off completely.*

Breathing deeply will help the recipient to relax.

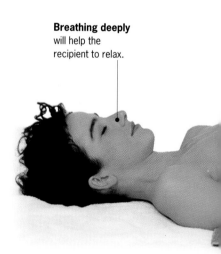

LIFESTYLE TIPS

▶ If you suffer regular cramps for no apparent reason, you might be lacking sufficient salt in your diet. Try increasing your salt intake slightly.

▶ If you have had a muscle spasm, it is important to rest afterward and allow the muscle to recover properly.

▶ Exercising regularly will help prevent cramps. Make sure that you warm up and cool down properly before and after working out.

3 Spasms in a foot can often affect the calf muscles as well. Taking the foot in one hand, gently knead the calf muscle up to the knee, working into the muscle with your fingertips. Repeat several times and ask the recipient to tell you if you are pressing too hard.

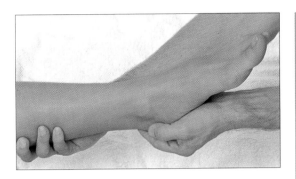

AROMATHERAPY

An antispasmodic essential oil can help relax muscles and prevent cramps.

▶ *Chamomile*

▶ *Lavender*

▶ *Rosemary**

*Rosemary should not be used by people who suffer from epilepsy.

Before using essential oils for massage, please read the information on safety and general use on pages 152–156.

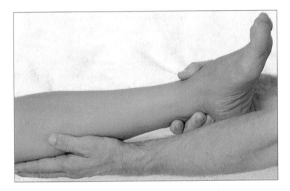

4 When you have finished kneading, stroke the muscle firmly to feel for any further tensions. If any exist, knead them further, using the technique in step 3. Stroking the lower leg helps improve blood circulation, which will stimulate a recovery response in the foot.

5 Firmly, and with both thumbs, apply circular thumb frictions between the bones of the foot from the toes toward the arch. Make sure that your thumbs move slowly and steadily with a moderate amount of pressure. Ask the recipient to tell you if the cramp is recurring at all. If so, start the massage again.

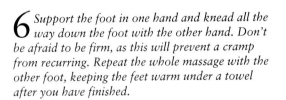

6 Support the foot in one hand and knead all the way down the foot with the other hand. Don't be afraid to be firm, as this will prevent a cramp from recurring. Repeat the whole massage with the other foot, keeping the feet warm under a towel after you have finished.

Muscles in the foot need to be fully relaxed after a spasm to prevent relapse.

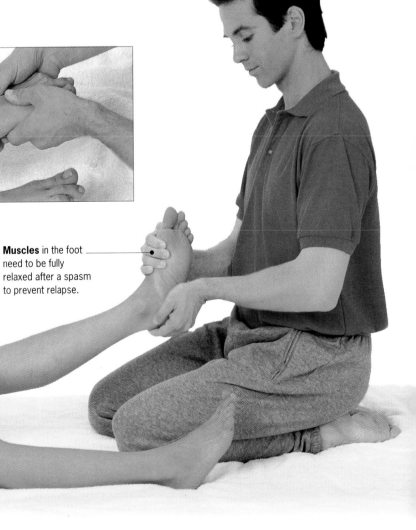

Arthritis in the Hands

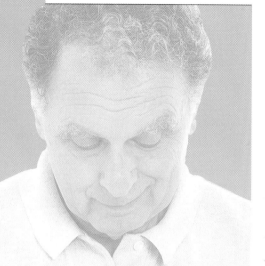

Anyone who is suffering from a painful and chronic condition such as arthritis can find support and emotional strength through a massage by a good friend or partner. However, in the more severe stages of arthritis, great care must be taken not to cause further damage, and massage should never be applied directly to an inflamed or extremely painful joint.

LIFESTYLE TIPS

▶ Taking it easy and feeling happy about yourself will improve your health. Don't try to carry on as usual when you feel unwell; you will become tired and down when you can't do everything you normally do.

▶ Exercise will relieve tension and ease joint mobility. Swimming is a very good therapy for arthritis because the water takes the weight off joints while the muscles are being exercised.

▶ Bathing in warm water will improve circulation, ease swelling, and relax muscles.

▶ Articulating a joint through its full range of movement will help loosen stiffness. However, do not stretch the joint if there is inflammation.

▶ Gently pull each finger away from the hand, outward, upward, and downward. Take each finger through its full range of movement.

▶ Finish the massage with a soothing stroke.

The stiffness of arthritis and the aches and pains associated with rheumatism can be eased with the use of simple massage techniques. Using massage every day will help loosen arthritic joints, particularly if it is started early in the development of the ailment. Most stiff joints will benefit from massage and stretching exercises, although this will depend on the type and severity of the arthritis. If the condition is in the acute phase, for example, if the joint is red, swollen, or excessively painful, massage must not be used and other treatment must be sought.

Rheumatism, a stiffness and achiness in the musculoskeletal system, is often seen as a prelude to arthritis. Rheumatoid arthritis is an acute condition in which the joints become inflamed and swollen. Stimulating the flow of lymph under the skin and between the joints can help ease the swelling and pain, because the waste products causing the swelling will be removed at a faster rate. The massage shown opposite can be used to ease stiff joints and soothe the related pain.

Arthritis in the hands can be both painful and debilitating. Make sure that the recipient is comfortable with the massage. Although a small amount of pain is to be expected, if it becomes uncomfortable, you must stop. If the recipient becomes restless, the benefits of the massage may be negated. It is often better to start a massage gently and then build up the pressure as you progress through it. This ensures that the recipient is given plenty of time to get used to the feelings of touch before any pressure is applied and can tell you if the procedure is painful. Keeping the recipient warm can increase relaxation; comfort is an important factor in all massage routines. You might be able to use the time to discuss any problems the recipient may have; many people who suffer from chronic conditions feel unable to voice their needs and may welcome an opportunity to talk.

CAUTION

People who suffer from arthritis must talk to their doctor before having massage treatment. Although it is of benefit in the early stages of the condition, during later stages massage can be detrimental to the joints. Also, if you are being massaged in any area affected by arthritis, tell the massager to stop immediately if you feel any pain. Positive benefits from massage will not be felt by a person who is hurting.

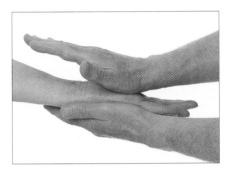

1 *Stroke the whole hand on both sides, from the wrist to the fingertips, and then push the heel of your hand along the front and back of the recipient's hand, moving back toward the wrist.*

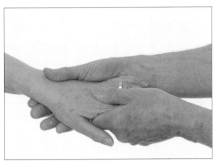

2 *Gently stroke around each joint and then carefully press your thumb around each joint with small circular motions. Keep the pressure as gentle and flowing as possible.*

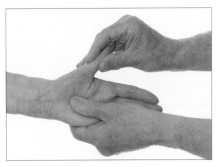

3 *Take the base of one thumb in your fingertips and gently roll it from side to side. Work your way up the thumb, paying particular attention to the joint, rolling gently. Repeat with the fingers and then work on the other hand.*

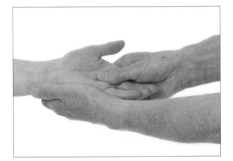

4 *With your thumb, press deeply into the palm, particularly the muscular area at the base of the thumb. Use small circular motions to relax the muscles.*

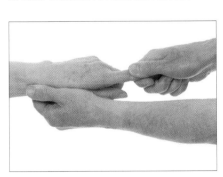

5 *Pull each finger gently away from the hand, outward, upward, and downward. Take each finger through its full range of movement.*

6 *Finish the massage with a soothing stroke over the whole hand, stroking each finger individually, then carefully massage it with an herbal moisturizer; this will help prevent chapping and keep the skin supple and smooth.*

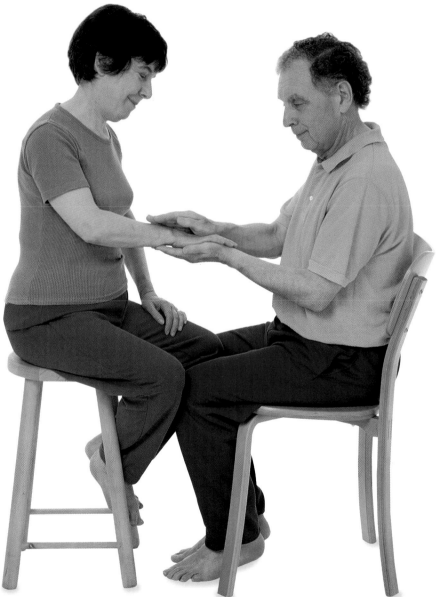

Headaches

One of the most common ailments, a headache is often caused by the tightening of muscles in the neck and scalp after periods of tension and stress. Eating problems, allergies, colds, flu, overwork, and alcohol and drug abuse can also produce headaches. Having someone give you a massage or doing it yourself can help ease the pain.

Although it is important to work on the entire head, focus the massage on the area where the pain is most acute. A head massage can be wonderfully relaxing, so try to sit or lie down quietly afterward and rest before doing anything demanding. The root cause of headaches is often stress. The headache itself might be telling you that you need to relax, so it is helpful to try to resolve the cause of the stress.

1 *Start the massage with a long, gentle stroke up the sides of the face, across the forehead, and through the hair to the nape of the neck. Repeat several times. This stimulates blood circulation through the area, which will hasten the recovery process and relieve any tension.*

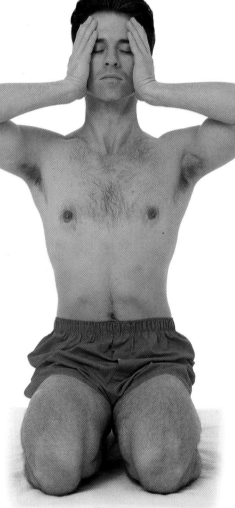

LIFESTYLE TIPS

▶ Taking time to relax regularly is essential if you are prone to headaches. Sitting with your eyes closed in a comfortable chair for 20 minutes every day can greatly reduce tension.

▶ Tension headaches can also be caused by a lack of sufficient sleep. Try to get a full night's sleep every night and avoid the use of sleep-inducing drugs.

▶ Make sure that your diet is well balanced and limit your intake of sugar and fat. Also, avoid an excessive intake of alcohol and caffeine.

TENSION HEADACHES

The tension headache is a common ailment. If you suffer frequently from such headaches, you can help yourself prevent them by practicing relaxation exercises. Relaxing through deep reflection (see page 38) or meditation (page 53) can give you the opportunity you need to recover from stress and stop tensions from building up. Yoga exercises and t'ai chi can also offer relief from pressure buildup.

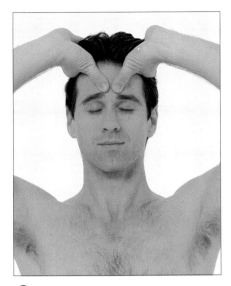

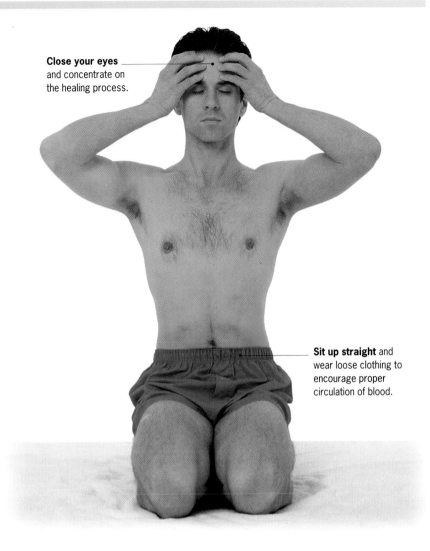

Close your eyes and concentrate on the healing process.

Sit up straight and wear loose clothing to encourage proper circulation of blood.

2 With your hands on your head, press your thumbs into the center of the forehead at the hairline. Press down the forehead to the top of the nose; repeat this action for several minutes.

3 Place the tips of your fingers together in the center of the forehead. Pressing firmly, draw your fingertips down each side of the face. Continue to work down your face, drawing your fingertips from the center outward and down the sides of your face and neck. Repeat several times.

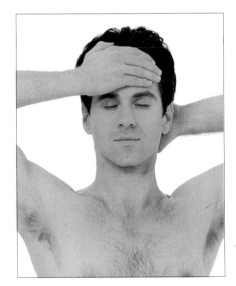

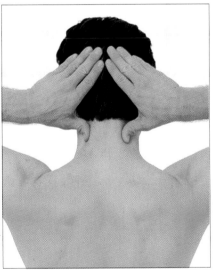

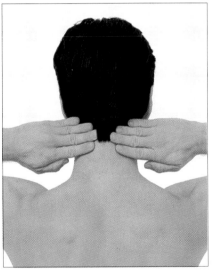

4 Place one hand on the back of the head and one hand on the forehead. Push on the forehead for 30 seconds.

5 With your thumbs, gently stroke up the back of the neck into the hair and repeat as many times as you wish.

6 Place the tips of your fingers at the base of the skull. From there, rotate them vigorously all over the scalp.

Depression

Depression can affect individuals in many different ways, and the symptoms are not always the same. Sufferers may feel a constant sadness, pessimism, or hopelessness, which can lead to a downward spiral of despair and isolation. Massage often relieves emotional pressures while the physical contact with another person brings comfort.

LIFESTYLE TIPS

▶ Exercising for 20 minutes or more will lift the spirits and help relieve the symptoms of depression. During exercise the body secretes chemicals—endorphins and enkephalins—into the bloodstream, which promote a feeling of well-being.

▶ Many emotional problems can be triggered or made worse by a diet that does not supply the body with all the essential nutrients. Make sure that your body is getting what it needs.

▶ Isolation is often associated with depression. Try not to cut yourself off from your friends and family; they will probably be more supportive and understanding than you think and will almost certainly be grateful that they have not been excluded from your life.

▶ Talking to others, or even writing down what you feel, can help you come to terms with your problems. Professional therapy is advised for serious or prolonged depression.

▶ Allow yourself plenty of time and opportunity to work through your depression.

Depression is frequently linked to deep anxiety in which a person finds it difficult to relax, possibly as a result of holding onto emotions such as anger, fear, resentment, or guilt. It can be very beneficial for a depressed person to talk about these feelings, although this may be hard to do. A full-body massage may be recommended, but people who are depressed often find it difficult to receive this type of massage, because they may feel particularly vulnerable in certain areas of the body. A face and head massage can be more appropriate, and the effect can be enhanced by the use of essential oils. There is no need for the recipient to undress, but clothing should be loose, especially around the neck area.

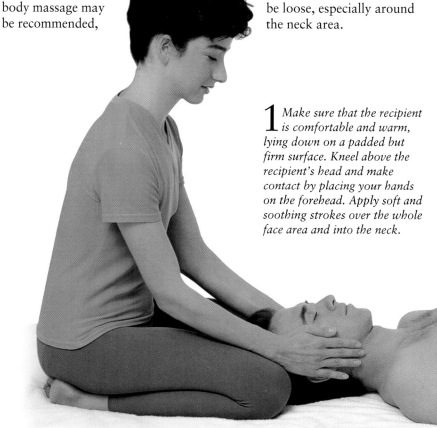

1 *Make sure that the recipient is comfortable and warm, lying down on a padded but firm surface. Kneel above the recipient's head and make contact by placing your hands on the forehead. Apply soft and soothing strokes over the whole face area and into the neck.*

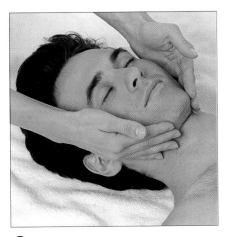

2 Beginning at the jawbone, use circular finger friction to massage all the areas of the face. Make sure that your strokes are slow and even to encourage relaxation.

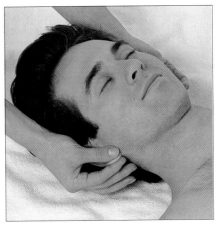

3 Take the ears between index fingers and thumbs and gently massage them, particularly the lobes. Starting from the top, pull them gently away from the head, working all the way down the edge.

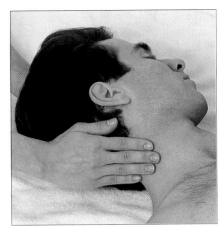

4 Turn the head to one side and, using the fingers, massage into the scalp area and the base of the head. Repeat on the other side, turning the head slowly and gently.

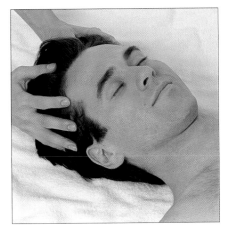

5 Using the fingertips, apply long and soothing strokes to the face and into the hair. This has a relieving effect and it may be a good opportunity for the recipient to share any problems.

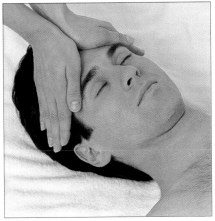

6 Finish by placing your hands lightly on the forehead. Ask the recipient to concentrate on breathing, taking deep, even breaths through the nose and breathing out through the mouth.

AROMATHERAPY

A number of essential oils are believed to have antidepressive properties, which can induce a feeling of well-being.

▶ Cedarwood

▶ Grapefruit

▶ Jasmine*

▶ Neroli

▶ Patchouli

▶ Rose*

▶ Ylang ylang

*Jasmine and rose should be avoided during pregnancy.

Before using essential oils for massage, please read the information on safety and general use given on pages 152–156.

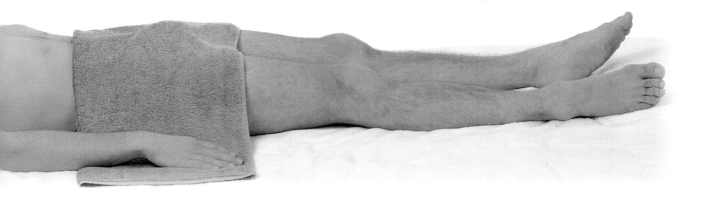

Neck and Shoulder Pain

If you've had a stressful day, have been sitting or standing improperly or carrying heavy loads, chances are that you have a buildup of tension in your neck and shoulders. This can cause you to hunch your shoulders and may lead to considerable pain. A neck and shoulder massage will release the tension, help you relax, and enable you to correct your posture.

The neck and shoulders bear the weight of the head and arms, which means they are in constant use from the time we get up in the morning until we go to bed at night. Carrying or moving heavy objects in an improper way can put extra strain on your shoulders and cause pain. Being conscious of your posture when carrying things or simply when sitting and standing will help you avoid aches and pains.

1 *Start the massage with a soothing stroke from the top of the neck down and over the shoulders. Outline the bones with your fingers, including those in the spine and in each shoulder. This can be deeply soothing and should be repeated several times. Ask the recipient to tell you where there are any areas of particular pain or tension.*

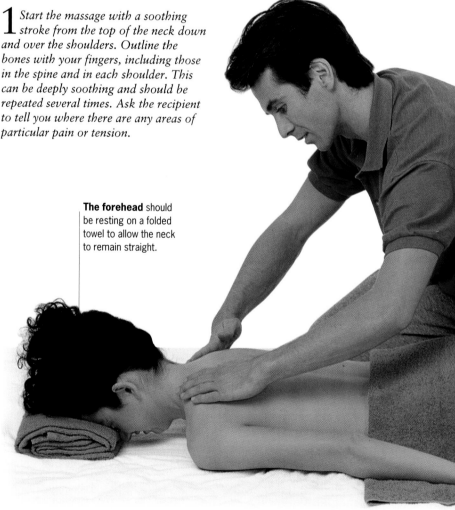

The forehead should be resting on a folded towel to allow the neck to remain straight.

LIFESTYLE TIPS

▶ Try to keep your posture upright and balanced at all times. If you are carrying heavy bags, do not slump or twist your body, and make sure that the weight is evenly distributed.

▶ Lying down helps the shoulder and neck areas to re-cover more quickly by relieving them of the weight of the head.

▶ Shoulder and neck pains are often caused by stress or by trying to do things too quickly. Think about what is making you stressed and try to minimize its effects.

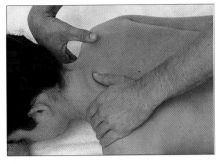

2 *Gently knead the tops of the shoulders and neck, gradually using stronger pressure to deal with the deeper muscle tensions.*

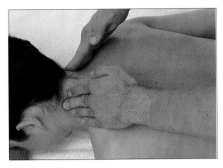

3 *Using your fingertips, apply circular pressure to the whole area. Try to etch out the shapes of the muscles and joints in small circular movements.*

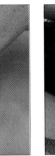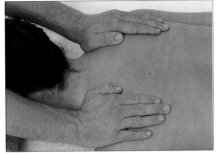

4 *With circular thumb movements, massage the upper backbone and up the neck. A great deal of tension can be stored here, so try to cover every joint.*

5 *Kneeling at the recipient's head, lay your hands on each shoulder and apply weight, asking how much pressure feels right. Hold for 2 minutes.*

6 *Finish the massage by gently pummeling the tops of the shoulders and upper back. Make sure that you cover the whole area. You can ask the recipient to say "AAAHHH" to help steady the breathing and enhance relaxation.*

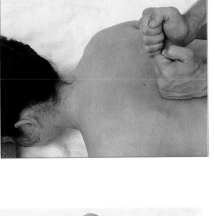

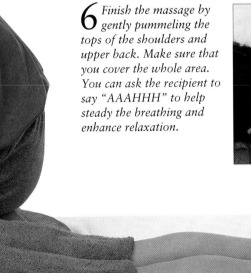

AROMATHERAPY

For soothing muscle pains and also relieving stress, the aromatherapy oils listed below can be very beneficial when used on a sore or stiff neck and shoulders. When the massage is finished, make a hot compress with a small towel and leave it over your neck and shoulders for 10 minutes.

▶ *Chamomile*

▶ *Frankincense**

▶ *Juniper**

▶ *Lavender*

▶ *Marjoram**

*Avoid during pregnancy.

Before using essential oils for massage, please read the information on safety and general use given on pages 152–156.

A WEIGHT OFF THE SHOULDERS

It is not a coincidence that we describe problems and worries as being a weight or burden on the shoulders: It has been proven that life's stresses often build up in the neck and shoulders, making us feel overloaded and heavy. Next time you feel tense, straighten your shoulders and stretch your neck upward; take a deep breath and relax. You will now be in a better state to cope with any problems. It can be helpful if you try not to take on too much at one time; overburdening yourself with work or worries is guaranteed to make you tense. Isolate each problem and seek a practical solution for it as soon as possible rather than letting problems build up and weigh you down.

Poor Circulation in the Legs

The average adult body contains approximately 5 liters (5 quarts) of blood, which transports vital nutrients and oxygen to all parts of the body. This is a constant and complex process, and it is important to sustain a steady rate at which blood travels around the system. The extremities, particularly the legs and feet, are the first places to suffer if blood circulation is poor.

The legs support the weight of the body and can collect a large amount of stress over time, especially if you work on your feet or spend a lot of time standing up. When massaging legs, never work over injuries or varicose veins. Anyone with a history of thrombosis should avoid leg massage.

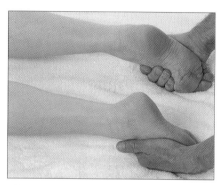

1 *With the recipient lying on his or her abdomen, make first contact by placing your hands under the feet. Take hold of a foot firmly in each hand, then place your hands over the soles, pressing gently but firmly and allowing your body heat to warm the skin.*

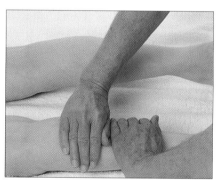

2 *Using both hands, apply your chosen oil to the leg, using long, even strokes up the leg and maintaining contact as the hands travel back down the leg to the foot. Ask the recipient to tell you if the pressure is uncomfortable. Always massage toward the heart, because this helps stimulate the circulation.*

LIFESTYLE TIPS

▶ Take up some form of aerobic exercise, like jogging, swimming, or brisk walking, for at least 20 minutes each day.

▶ Maintain a healthy and balanced diet to prevent sluggish circulation. Try cutting down on fats and eating more fresh fruits and vegetables.

▶ Poor circulation is linked with stress, as are heart conditions. Taking time to relax regularly and work through your problems will improve your general health.

CIRCULATION TIPS

▶ *Invest in a body brush and brush the skin briskly every day, always brushing toward the heart.*

▶ *As you finish showering, turn the water to cold for about 30 seconds. Cold water can get the blood flowing.*

▶ *Spend 10 minutes every day lying down with your legs and feet raised above waist level.*

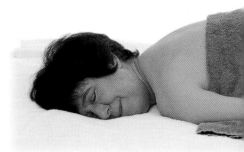

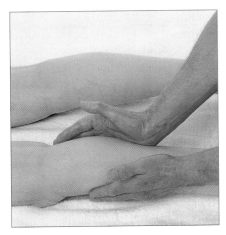

3 *Apply kneading movements to the calf, working upward and into the thighs. This helps the blood flow faster through the tissues of the skin and muscles and produces a warming effect. It is also good for the skin, enhancing its condition and self-cleansing qualities.*

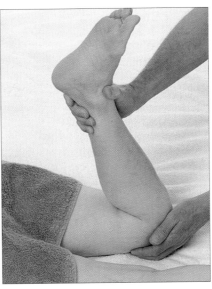

4 *Lift the foot and lower leg and bend the knee to its full extent. Repeat several times, speeding up the movement slightly to stimulate blood flow and improve flexibility in the knee joints.*

AROMATHERAPY

A number of essential oils stimulate the circulation. The first three listed below are rubefacients, which create warmth and redness.

▶ *Black pepper*

▶ *Ginger*

▶ *Rosemary* *

▶ *Frankincense* †

▶ *Juniper* †

*Rosemary should not be used by people who have epilepsy.

† Avoid frankincense and juniper during pregnancy.

Before using essential oils for massage, please read the information on safety and general use given on pages 152–156.

5 *With your hands parallel to each other, pummel up and down the back of each leg twice. Ask the recipient to tell you if you are pummeling too hard and take special care around the ankle, where the ligament can easily be damaged by pressure.*

6 *Take a foot in each hand and gently shake the legs. You don't have to lift them off the floor, just move them slowly from side to side. When you have finished shaking the legs, close the massage by holding the feet firmly in your hands.*

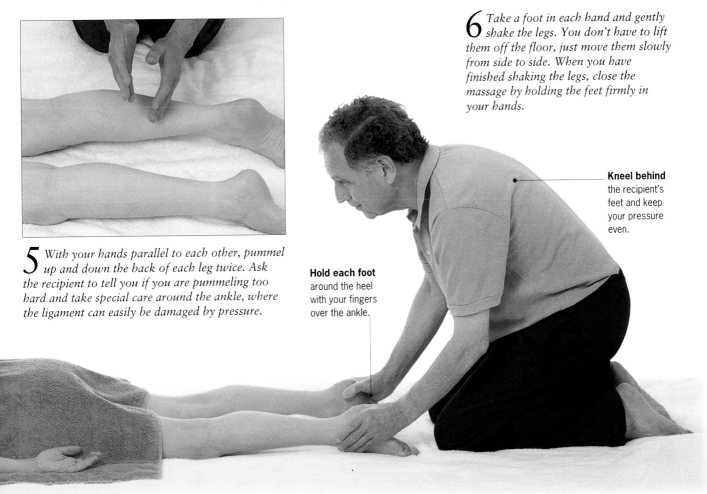

Kneel behind the recipient's feet and keep your pressure even.

Hold each foot around the heel with your fingers over the ankle.

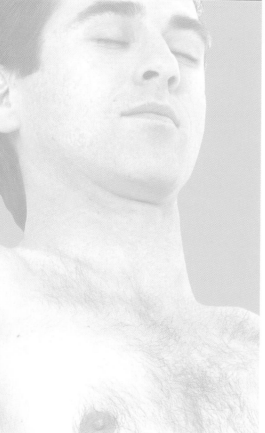

Constipation

A common condition, constipation occurs when the body has difficulty in expelling the waste products of digestion. It can cause discomfort and pain and may also lead to a number of more serious complaints. A variety of factors can bring on constipation, including poor diet, a lazy bowel, lack of sufficient exercise, and emotional problems such as insecurity or anxiety.

Massage can be an excellent way to improve the functioning of your bowels, although you must make sure that any other factors that may be causing constipation, for example, poor diet or lack of exercise, are also being dealt with. The massage can be done by someone else, or you can do it yourself, which may be more effective because you can judge the response better and adapt the massage to your own needs. If constipation continues after you have tried massage, made changes to your diet, and increased your exercise, you should seek professional advice. There may be a more serious problem, such as an ulcer, irritable bowel syndrome, or cancer.

A massage eases the passage of waste matter by stimulating the colon, or large intestine. Do not press too hard because you may damage the colon if the blockage is severe. If there is considerable tension in the abdomen, begin by feeling around to locate the colon, small intestine, and, for a woman, the reproductive organs. Sometimes constipation is caused by more major disorders, so also feel for any abnormalities or swellings, such as in the appendix on the lower right side of the abdomen, or in the ovaries. If there is any cause for concern, consult a doctor.

Be careful not to damage the intestines when you massage; using many gentle strokes is far better than a few strong ones. A hot-water bottle or heating pad can often ease any discomfort and promote movement through the gut.

LIFESTYLE TIPS

▶ Take time to let your body function properly. When you feel a bowel movement coming, make a point of stopping everything else to accommodate it; give it top priority.

▶ Make sure that your diet is high in fiber, found in whole grains, fruits, and vegetables.

▶ Consider your emotional state and your lifestyle. Ask yourself if there are any factors that are causing you anxiety or insecurity and how these can be alleviated.

▶ Increase your exercise; it will speed up your body's functions, including elimination of waste.

A BALANCED DIET

In traditional Chinese medicine, a balanced diet comprises a mixture of yin and yang foods. It is thought to play an important role in keeping the intestines and the whole body in good general health by bringing the opposite forces into equilibrium within the system. Yin foods include milk, bread, and chicken, whereas red meat and chilies are yang foods.

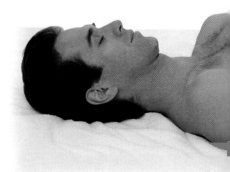

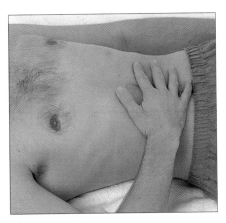

1 *Feel for the colon running up the right side of the abdomen, across the waist, and down the left side. Try to feel the shape and locate where blockages might be occurring.*

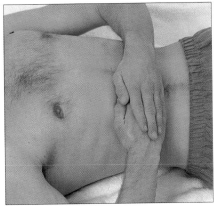

2 *Gently stroke clockwise around the colon—the direction of the bowel movement. At first, use light strokes, getting firmer as you progress but never using hard pressure. Constipation is often associated with the buildup of air pockets within the system, and if there should be any, putting pressure on these areas can strain the intestines.*

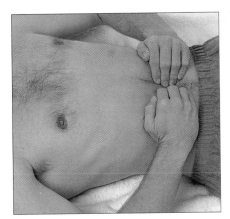

3 *Starting on the right side, gently knead your way up the colon. Knead across the center, just beneath your waist, and down the left side.*

4 *Place one hand over the other and press with small circular movements around the colon, taking deep, long breaths as you massage.*

5 *Place your hands on opposite sides of the abdomen and gently pull them together so they pass in the middle, then stroke down your sides. Repeat several times.*

Movements
should be gentle
and flowing.

AROMATHERAPY

Aromatherapy can help stimulate the muscle action that aids the digestive activity and the evacuation of the bowels. The following can be used in massage oils.

► *Fennel**

► *Ginger*

► *Lemongrass*

► *Mandarin*

► *Orange*

► *Rosemary †*

* Avoid fennel during pregnancy.

† Rosemary should not be used by people who have epilepsy.

Before using essential oils for massage, please read the information on safety and general use given on pages 152–156.

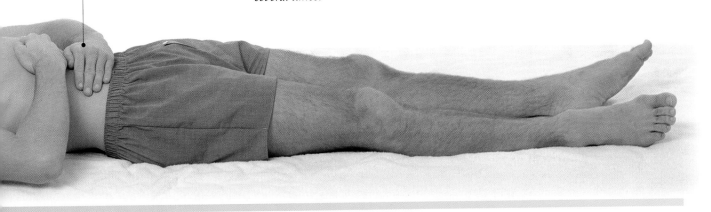

Breathing Problems

Tightness in the chest is usually caused by asthma or bronchitis. Asthma can be triggered by a number of factors, from anxiety to allergies caused by airborne substances, while bronchitis is an inflammation of the air tubes and is indicated by a wheezing cough. Massage can help clear the air passages and relax the throat, allowing for easier breathing and relaxation.

Easing the lung muscles and reducing the levels of general stress are the priorities when massaging a person suffering from bronchitis or asthma. Chest and back massage will help to open the chest area. However, these are both serious conditions that need professional medical care for overall management. If the recipient is a woman, do not massage over the breasts but work around them.

Before starting the massage, ask the recipient to take five or six deep breaths, holding the air in the lungs for a few seconds. This will begin relaxation and loosen up the muscles in the chest area. Ask the recipient to tell you about any particular soreness or problem areas so that you can focus on them during the massage.

Start the massage by placing your warmed hands on the chest to make initial contact and calm the patient. The massage normally takes 15 to 20 minutes, although you should continue massaging until the recipient can breathe easily and is relaxed and calm. Some of the massage strokes help to loosen phlegm from the breathing channels and lungs, and these should be repeated if the recipient has difficulty clearing the breathing passages. Be gentle with any tender spots; pain or soreness may cause the recipient to constrict the chest muscles.

LIFESTYLE TIPS

▶ Regular exercise can both relax and strengthen the lungs. However, if you have an allergy to an airborne substance, such as pollen, make sure you are not breathing it in while exercising. Swimming is a good exercise for asthmatics.

▶ Contact with any known allergens should be reduced or, if possible, completely avoided.

▶ Relaxing and not panicking will ease breathing problems. It is essential to try to keep calm during an asthma attack.

ACUPRESSURE

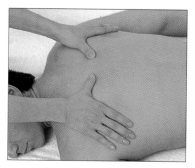

BLADDER 13 – THE LUNG POINT
Two finger widths out from the spine at the third vertebra from the base of the neck, press for 2 minutes to ease breathing problems.

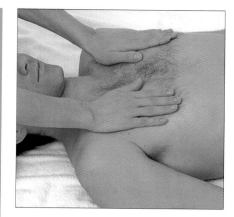

1 *Kneeling behind the recipient's head, make contact by placing your hands on the center of the chest. Both of you should focus on breathing deeply and evenly and making sure that you are completely relaxed.*

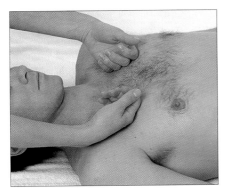

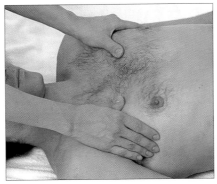

2 *Apply finger or knuckle rotations under the collarbone and into the shoulder joints. Repeat this action, using the thumbs but taking care not to exert so much pressure that the recipient feels discomfort.*

3 *Using the thumbs, apply thumb frictions from the center of the chest out to the sides, working on the muscles between the ribs. Use the thumbs to stretch these muscles, always working from the center to the sides of the body.*

4 *With your hands loosely clasped, very gently pummel the chest area of the recipient. Ask him or her to make a low "AAAHHH" sound as you pummel. This will help release any phlegm from the chest and throat areas.*

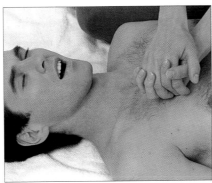

AROMATHERAPY

Although not intended to replace orthodox treatment for asthma, the aromatherapy oils below can help by soothing inflammation and reducing muscle spasms. They can also improve breathing. Inhalations of oils should not be used in cases of asthma or bronchitis, as they can further irritate already inflamed mucous membranes and could bring on an attack.

► *Chamomile*
► *Cypress**
► *Eucalyptus*
► *Lavender*
► *Marjoram**
► *Rose**
► *Valerian†*

*Avoid cypress, marjoram, and rose during pregnancy.

†Valerian is a strong sedative, and you must avoid using machinery after treatment.

Before using essential oils for massage, please read the information on safety and general use given on pages 152–156.

5 *Finish with gentle, soothing strokes, using the tips of the fingers over the lung area. Both of you should be concentrating on regular, deep breathing and enjoying the relaxation.*

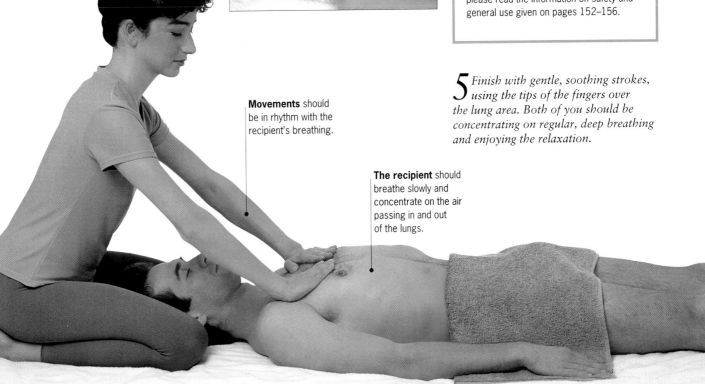

Movements should be in rhythm with the recipient's breathing.

The recipient should breathe slowly and concentrate on the air passing in and out of the lungs.

Tension in the Back

Back problems, often accompanied by acute aches and pains, can be triggered by a number of factors, including bad posture, poor lifting techniques, the buildup of tension in the muscles, or an injury. A soothing back massage will not necessarily cure the problem, but it will certainly be welcomed for its muscle-relaxing effects.

Bad posture, both in sitting and standing, is one of the main causes of back trouble, which can largely be avoided by remembering to keep your neck and shoulders upright and your backbone straight. Doing stretching exercises occasionally will ease any buildup of tension. If you are lifting a heavy object, do not twist your body or stoop to pick it up, as this places strain on the back. Instead, crouch down and lift by straightening your legs so that they take the weight, not your back.

LIFESTYLE TIPS

▶ Many exercises are good for preventing back problems. One of these is yoga (see page 56). Swimming and other exercises in water can help ease back pain (see pages 72–73).

▶ Pay close attention to your posture and lifting techniques. If you are carrying more than one bag, make sure that the weight is evenly distributed.

▶ Relaxation is one of the keys to recovery from back trouble. Try breathing exercises, yoga, or meditation, and make sure that you get plenty of sleep.

▶ Monitor which parts of your life are most stressful and think of ways to avoid or reduce the stress factors.

▶ If you are going through a particularly stressful period, limit or, better still, avoid coffee, alcohol, and smoking, which can increase tension.

1 *With the recipient lying on his or her abdomen, kneel to one side of the body. Place one hand on the nape of the neck and the other at the base of the spine and hold for a few moments, breathing deeply and feeling the connection between the two of you. Apply massage oil to the whole back and buttocks in long, flowing, and soothing strokes. Repeat the strokes several times.*

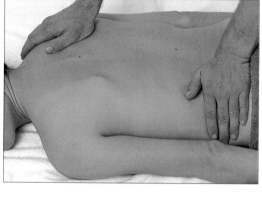

MUSCLE STRAIN

Most back pain is a result of muscle strain, which occurs when the muscle fibers are torn or stretched from being pulled too far or overworked. The torn muscle fibers bleed into the surrounding area or muscle, causing pain, swelling, and muscle spasm. Strained muscles will heal themselves with time, although recovery can be speeded up by certain physiotherapy techniques.

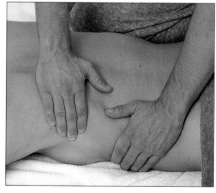

2 *Using both hands, apply kneading movements all the way up each side of the back. Press into the shoulders and knead the top of the arms. Repeat a second time, increasing the pressure.*

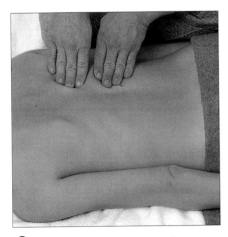

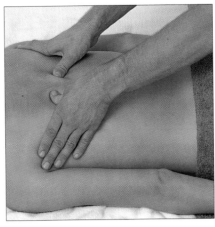

3 *Using the fingers held closely together and working up one side of the back, apply circular movements to spinal muscles. Try to etch the outside of each bone in the spine to ease tension out of the muscles. Repeat on the other side.*

4 *Using circular movements with the thumbs, work up the back on either side of the spine, around the shoulders, and into the neck. Pay special attention to areas that feel lumpy or tight, checking the pressure with the recipient.*

AROMATHERAPY

A number of essential oils are sedative in nature and so can calm both body and mind. It may be beneficial to burn some essential oils and encourage a massage recipient to breathe deeply and evenly. Counting breaths can help people who are tense become calmer.

▶ *Bergamot*
▶ *Chamomile*
▶ *Lavender*
▶ *Neroli, or orange blossom*
▶ *Rose**
▶ *Sandalwood*

*Avoid during pregnancy.

Before using essential oils for massage, please read the information on safety and general use given on pages 152–156.

5 *Straighten the recipient's neck by resting her forehead on a folded towel. Gently apply kneading motions to the back of the neck and into the base of the skull. The neck muscles carry a lot of stress, so repeat several times.*

6 *Using the tips of your fingers, do feather-light strokes down the recipient's back. Finish the massage by resting your hands on the upper back with a gentle pressure for a few moments.*

Cover the part of the body not being massaged.

Knead well around the shoulder blades to improve mobility.

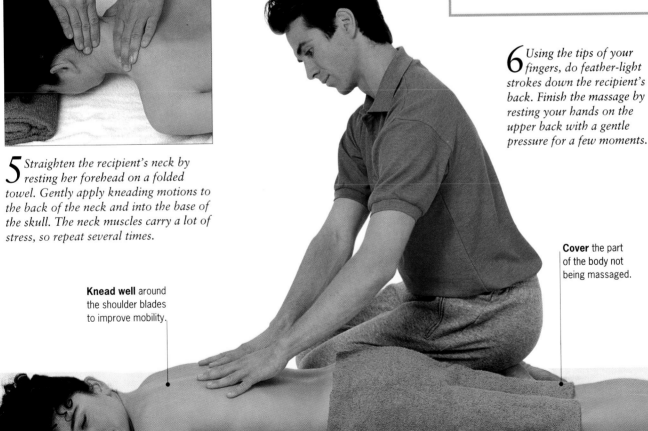

Massage for the Elderly

Feeling happy and positive about growing older is one of the greatest health boosts possible for the elderly. Massage can help alleviate stiffness, stimulate circulation, and improve the immune system, enhancing all-round physical health. It doesn't matter how old the recipient is, a gentle massage can promote good health and a feeling of well-being in everyone.

It is important that an older person feel relaxed and at ease with a massage, especially if he or she is frail. The massage described below is informal, with the recipient sitting on an upright chair, such as the one pictured opposite, and fully clothed. This approach makes it possible to perform the massage in a variety of situations and with little preparation. Any of the massages shown on pages 104–123 can also be given to the elderly, but you must be gentle and considerate of the recipient's physical health, asking if there are any problem areas that need to be avoided.

pages 104–123

LIFESTYLE TIPS

▶ Older people should increase their intake of fresh fruits and vegetables so that they are obtaining a good balance of vitamins and minerals.

▶ Exercise will rebalance the impact of aging on muscles. Good options include swimming, cycling, and walking briskly.

▶ Relaxation techniques will improve a person's health and state of mind. They are also good for dealing with stress and chronic pain.

▶ A hobby can renew interest in life and thus enhance health and well-being.

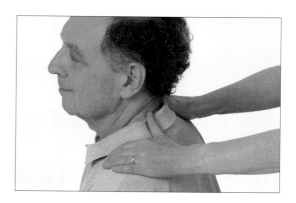

1 *With the recipient sitting comfortably on an upright chair, gently massage the shoulders until both of you feel relaxed and comfortable. It may help if you talk to each other, or you might ask if the patient has any areas of weakness or pain that would benefit from special attention.*

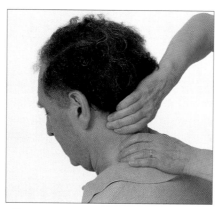

2 *Gently massage the back of the neck using light stroking actions with the fingertips. Move your fingers around the neck to the front and then back again.*

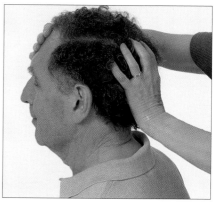

3 *Place one hand firmly on the forehead and gently massage the back of the head and the neck area with the other hand.*

4 *Holding the back of the head with one hand, gently massage the forehead with the other, using small circular movements with your fingertips. After a minute you can increase the pressure, although you should check with the recipient first.*

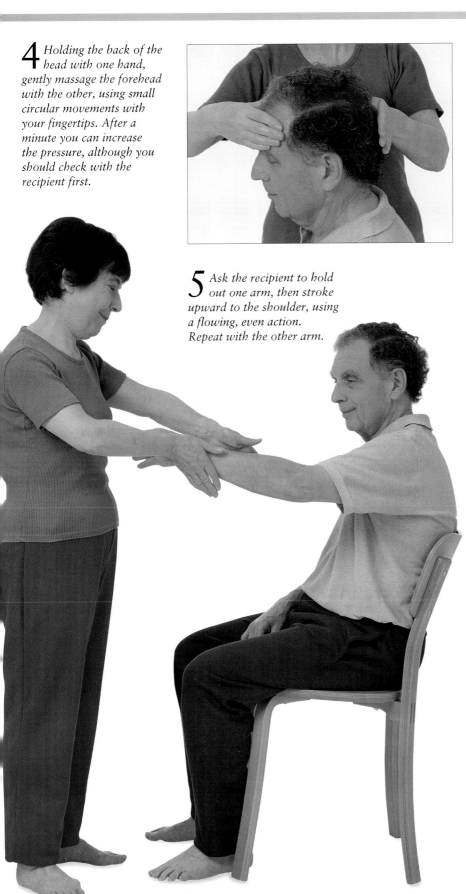

5 *Ask the recipient to hold out one arm, then stroke upward to the shoulder, using a flowing, even action. Repeat with the other arm.*

YOU ARE ONLY AS OLD AS YOU FEEL

It is difficult to define the term *elderly* in regard to years; what is diminished old age for one person is a full and active life for another. It has been suggested by many alternative therapists that people become old when they feel they have nothing left to live for, possibly because of the death of those close to them, or when they feel they have lived too long already. People who retain their health well into old age are those who are still open to new ideas and making a fresh start with new friends and hobbies.

The relief of worries and stresses through massage can encourage good health and a feeling of well-being. Many older people have a need to be touched, particularly if they live on their own, in order to feel in contact with the outer world. This can be an important step toward a sense of worth, friendship, and relaxation.

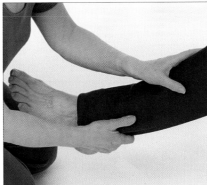

6 *Taking hold of the back of the ankle, stroke up the leg to above the knee. Repeat several times, then do the same stroke on the other leg. This greatly improves blood circulation in the legs and feet, which can be beneficial for the health of the elderly and the weak.*

Massage for Couples

A healthy relationship requires good communication, and body contact is one of the most intimate and powerful communication tools we possess. Touch through massage is an excellent way to relax the body, invoke deep emotional feelings, and reinforce feelings of love and togetherness. Couples can also use massage to help overcome sexual problems.

Sex is the most intimate and vulnerable act of affection, when two people become extremely open to each other and allow their bodies to experience the ecstasy of orgasm. Sometimes, however, difficulties arise in relationships that inhibit openness and trust. Problems can include fears about sexual prowess, negative associations with sex, feelings of isolation during lovemaking, or not being able to connect with a partner. Any of these can lead to anxiety and affect an individual's response to making love, sometimes resulting in lack of libido, impotence, or frigidity. Sex is a physical activity, and it is important to be physically relaxed and comfortable to avoid mental chatter, which can ruin the moment.

When a couple is having difficulties with sexual contact, the pair might benefit from an informal massage technique known as sensate focus. This will help them get in touch with each other and discover the pleasurable sensations involved in intimate physical contact.

Sensate focus involves the couple putting aside at least two 1-hour sessions every week to relax with each other. Based on easy massage techniques and caressing, the first 10 sessions are limited to nonsexual areas of the body. The stimulation of erotic areas of the body, and eventually the genitals, is gradually introduced when both partners feel comfortable and relaxed. It is important that the couple not have sexual intercourse during the early stages of the course but wait until the exploration and feedback from the process of massage without sex is complete. Communication is one of the biggest problems concerning sexual difficulties, and learning to respond to physical touch and stimulation can be one of the most important barriers to break. Massage can help two people cross these boundaries, opening the way toward a more caring and understanding relationship. It can help individuals rediscover the pleasures and sensations of being close to someone special and sharing a healthy sex life.

ACUPRESSURE

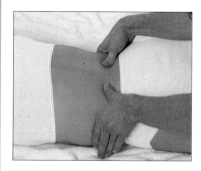

BLADDER 23 – THE KIDNEY POINT
Two finger widths from the spine, just below the waist, press for 2 minutes to increase sexual drive.

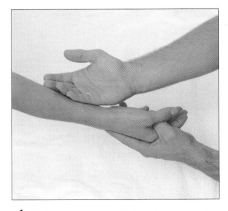

1 *Take your partner's hand and gently massage the fingers and stroke the palm. Then lift the arm away from the body and run your hand up the arm and onto the shoulder. Do this several times, then repeat with the other arm.*

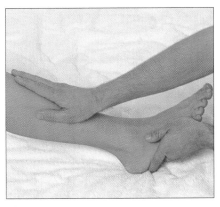

2 *Squeeze the foot gently between your hands and stroke up the leg, keeping a steady and flowing movement to foster relaxation. Repeat the same movements on the other leg.*

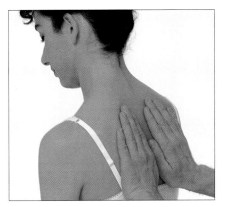

3 *With your partner sitting in front of you, gently stroke the back, running both hands up the spine and neck and pushing your fingers into the hair. Run your hands back down your partner's sides and then repeat.*

4 *With your partner sitting in front of you, gently massage the neck. First, run your fingers up the back of the neck and then up the sides and front. Next, starting at the front, stroke gently downward and repeat this around the neck to the back.*

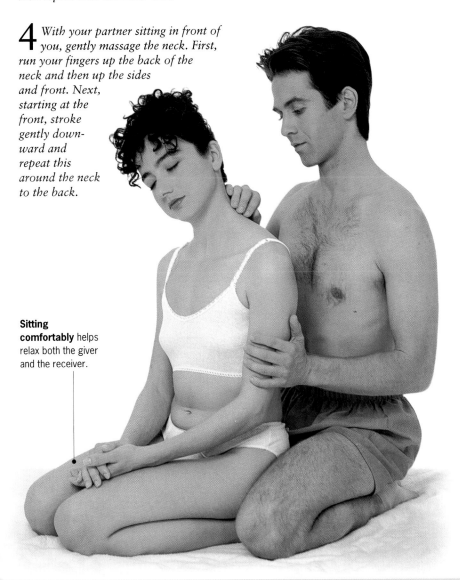

Sitting comfortably helps relax both the giver and the receiver.

AROMATHERAPY

A number of oils are classified as aphrodisiacs and can be excellent for inducing a romantic and sensual atmosphere. In the following list, the first five are woody, sensuous, and earthy aphrodisiac oils with a grounding quality that helps take the focus away from the mind and bring it to the body, warming and relaxing it. The last three are romantic oils that can create a sense of sacredness and reinforce the bond between lovers.

▶ *Cedarwood*

▶ *Damiana*

▶ *Patchouli*

▶ *Sandalwood*

▶ *Vetiver*

▶ *Jasmine**

▶ *Rose**

▶ *Ylang ylang*

*Avoid during pregnancy.

Before using essential oils for massage, please read the information on safety and general use given on pages 152–156.

Menstrual Pains

Most women suffer from some kind of menstrual discomfort—commonly, cramps in the uterus and abdomen during the first days of the period. Menstrual pain may be a dull ache, or it can be severe cramping that encompasses the whole abdomen. Massage can alleviate period pains, especially when used in combination with aromatherapy massage oils.

One of the most natural reactions to abdominal pain is to curl up somewhere warm and lie still until the pain goes away. However, it is often better to give yourself a good massage, stretching the muscles and allowing your body to work through the muscle movements.

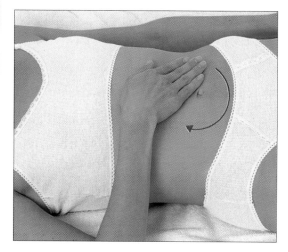

1 *Lie on your back with a cushion under both knees so that your back is flat against the floor or bed. Apply massage oil in clockwise, circular, soothing strokes following the route of the colon, or large intestine, up the right side of the abdomen, across the top, and down the left side. Repeat several times.*

LIFESTYLE TIPS

▶ A connection has been found between diet and painful periods. Try to avoid alcohol, coffee, dairy products, and foods made with refined starches and sugars a few days before and during your period.

▶ Chamomile is an anti-spasmodic, and drinking plenty of chamomile tea can help release muscle tension. This will also generally relax and calm the body and mind.

▶ It is recommended, whenever possible, to keep stress to a minimum during your period. It can be beneficial to plan some time for rest and relaxation during this time.

2 *Place both hands below your ribs with fingers meeting in the middle and apply firm strokes from the center outward. Repeat six times.*

Use small, gentle strokes, especially over the lower abdomen.

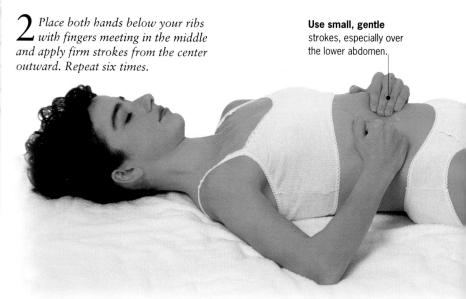

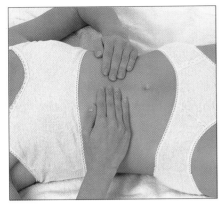

3 *Move your fingers in circular movements below the ribs, working from the center out to the sides of the abdomen. This helps to settle the entire stomach and abdominal area.*

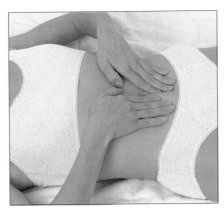

4 *Place your hands over the lower abdomen, where the uterus sits, and very gently stroke upward and out to the sides. Repeat these movements several times in a soothing, rhythmic flow.*

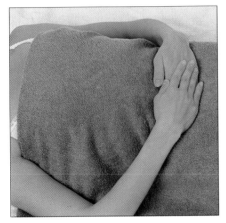

5 *Finish by covering yourself to keep warm, then lay your hands on the lower abdomen or on the spot where there is pain. Let the hands gently rest there and warm the area. As you do this, take slow, deep breaths.*

ACUPRESSURE

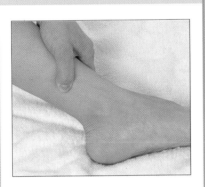

SPLEEN 6
Pressing Spleen 6, four finger widths above the anklebone, can relieve period pains. Press for 2 minutes. Avoid during pregnancy.

AROMATHERAPY

Aromatherapy can be very useful in easing menstrual pains. It can be used in a number of ways, from massaging the abdomen and applying a compress to using the oils in a luxurious long bath. Because menstrual pains are often due to muscle spasm, antispasmodic oils are chosen.

► *Chamomile*
► *Clary sage**‡*
► *Frankincense**
► *Juniper**
► *Lavender*
► *Rose**
► *Valerian†*

Rose carries with it many associations with femininity and is considered the queen of the essential oils. It is a luxurious, if costly, oil and is used to create an uplifting mood.

Juniper and frankincense are diuretics and can therefore be used to help the body reduce fluid retention.

Aromatherapy can also be very beneficial for premenstrual syndrome, helping to balance the body's hormones. Some oils are emmenagogues; that is, they can induce menstrual bleeding and rebalance the hormonal system. Two in particular are rose and frankincense.

* Avoid clary sage, frankincense, juniper, and rose during pregnancy, because there is evidence that they may cause miscarriage.

‡ Avoid alcohol when using clary sage.

† Valerian essential oil has very powerful sedative properties, and it is better to rest for a while after using it.

Before using essential oils for massage, please read the information on safety and general use given on pages 152–156.

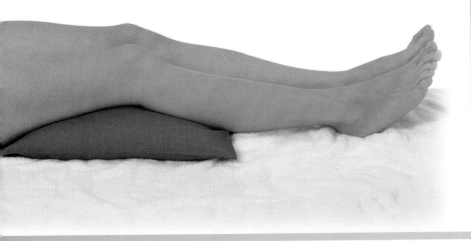

Relaxing Body Massage

Most people suffer from restlessness or insomnia during some period in their lives, leaving them feeling tired, stressed, and unable to function properly. Insomnia can be caused by a number of factors, including allergies, a poor diet, illness, or stress. Massage can promote relaxation, allowing the mind to forget the troubles of the day and relax into sleep.

Relaxation is one key to resolving insomnia. Massage helps an insomniac calm down and stop thinking about minor worries. It can also ease aches and pains and pave the way for comfortable sleep. The massage should be firm, even rough at times. The idea is to exhaust the recipient, who should not be asked to do anything before, during, or after massage.

INSOMNIA

If you are having trouble sleeping, eliminate as many external stimuli as possible. Reducing light and noise and making sure that the room temperature is comfortable are the first steps to ensuring relaxation and sound sleep.

LIFESTYLE TIPS

► If you are kept awake by worries, make a list of your problems and vow to think about them in the morning. Putting them aside will help you relax and sleep.

► Relaxation techniques, such as quiet reflection (page 38), a long warm bath (page 35), or meditation (page 53), can be excellent remedies for sleeping problems.

► Sometimes people can't sleep because they are not physically tired, even though their brains are exhausted. Make sure that you get enough physical activity every day.

1 *Start by stroking the entire body, from the feet all the way to the top of the head, using your whole hands either together or separately. Keep movements fluid. If you can't reach from the feet to the head in one movement, use sweeping actions up the body until you have covered the body completely.*

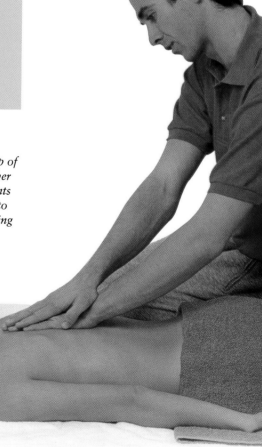

2 The shoulders are particularly susceptible to muscle tension. Give them a firm kneading to release deeper tensions. Using each hand alternately, lift the skin of the shoulders, pushing your thumbs into the muscles. Do not be afraid to be firm; harder pressure will induce drowsiness so that the recipient will be ready for sleep afterward.

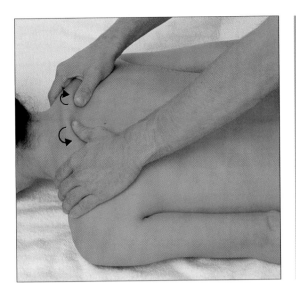

AROMATHERAPY

There are a number of sedative oils that can counter restlessness and insomnia and induce a restful state.

▶ *Bergamot*

▶ *Chamomile*

▶ *Lavender*

▶ *Neroli*

▶ *Sandalwood*

Before using essential oils for massage, please read the information on safety and general use given on pages 152–156.

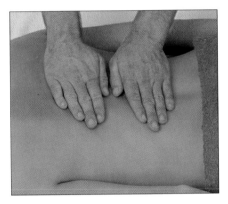

3 Place your hands next to each other at the base of the back and firmly push the heels into the muscles on the side of the spine closest to you. Work up to the neck and into the hair. Repeat several times and then do the other side.

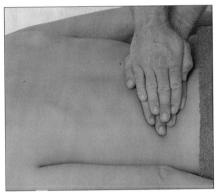

4 Place your hands together in the middle of the back. Put some of your weight onto the back and hold for 2 minutes—enough to allow the recipient to feel slightly uncomfortable. Repeat.

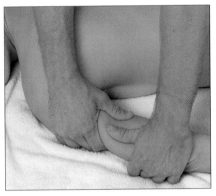

5 Firmly knead the arms and neck. You can use a kneading action and a squeezing action alternately. When squeezing, use both hands together and work up the arm. After you have finished, shake the arm firmly.

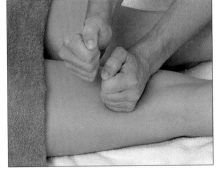

6 The legs carry the weight of the body and may hold a lot of tension. Starting at the top, pummel down each leg. Be firm; you want to feel all the tension released from the recipient.

Drape the recipient with towels for warmth.

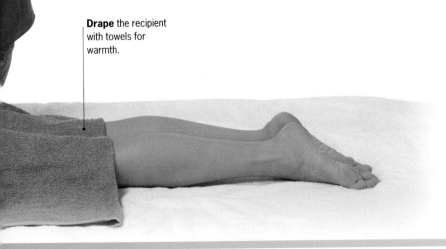

Massage for Pregnancy

A gentle massage during pregnancy can uplift the mother and settle the baby, easing away stresses and tensions. It can also relieve other problems that are associated with pregnancy, such as backache, insomnia, anxiety, and digestive disorders. However, several aromatherapy oils must be avoided: see pages 154–155 or consult a trained aromatherapist.

Self-massage during pregnancy relieves stress and promotes good health for you and your baby. Because it is important not to put stress on the baby, you should use only soft stroking actions, never any fast or jerky movements. Avoid all pummeling and percussion methods.

Massage can also be given by a friend or partner. A good back, shoulder, and neck massage can be done with the mother-to-be sitting astride an upright chair and leaning forward on the back of it. (Techniques can be adapted from those on pages 122–125.) Many women also benefit greatly from a soothing neck and shoulder massage during labor; it helps them relax and feel supported, especially if labor is prolonged.

> **WARNING**
> *Care must be taken when massaging the abdomen of a pregnant woman, especially during the first 12 weeks of pregnancy, when the risk of miscarriage is highest. Be gentle and avoid direct pressure. Also, avoid certain aromatherapy oils.*

1 *Gently stroke the contours of your abdomen, feeling the shape of the embryonic sac. First use your fingertips and then, still very gently, use your whole hand.*

LIFESTYLE TIPS

▶ It is important to set aside periods for relaxation during pregnancy, preserving your energy to help the fetus develop and to prepare for childbirth.

▶ Make a conscious effort to reduce the stresses in your life. You may find that problems overwhelm you quickly and it requires great effort to deal with even small crises.

▶ Make sure that your diet provides all the essential nutrients you need for your own health and the development of the baby. Eating calcium-rich foods is especially important.

Never put pressure directly on the abdomen.

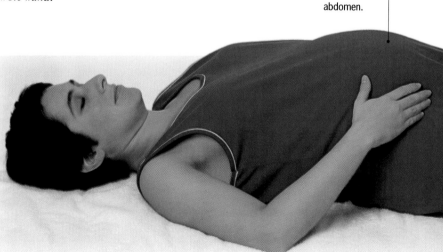

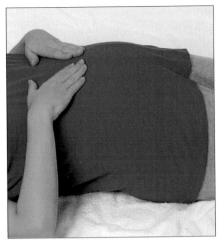

2 Stroke clockwise around the navel, starting small and moving your hands in a larger circle until you have covered the whole stomach area.

3 With a hand on each side, stroke from the sides of the stomach to the center. Use long, flowing strokes and take your time; the strokes should be slow and even. Try to breathe deeply at the same pace as your strokes; this will enhance relaxation and allow the soothing rhythm to penetrate the womb. Repeat several times. This may be a good opportunity for you to think about the baby's needs, contemplating your diet and general health and fitness.

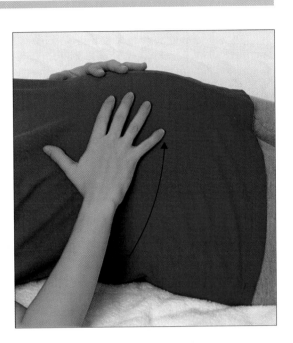

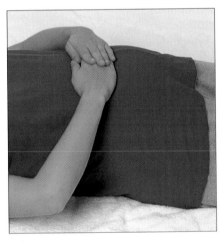

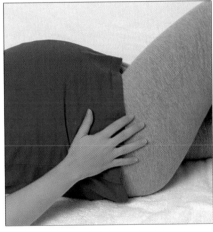

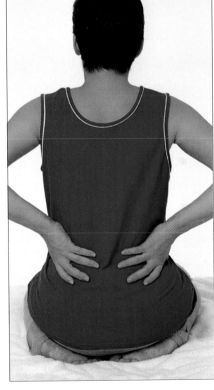

4 With one hand on top of the other and flat on your body, stroke up the abdomen to the chest and then back down, covering the whole stomach area.

5 With your right leg bent, massage the top of your thigh and hip using small circular movements and pressing into the muscles. Repeat on the left side.

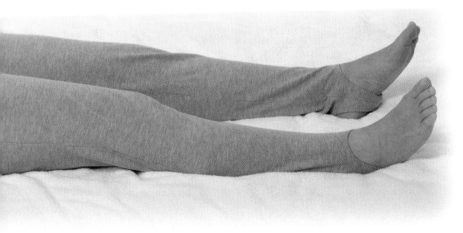

6 Finish the massage kneeling upright and stroking down your lower back. The lower back takes a great deal of the strain when you are pregnant, so spend some time on this area. Find the pockets of tension and ease them out, using slow, firm strokes with the pressure coming from your palm.

Massage for Children

Touching and stroking babies and children is beneficial to their development, and many health specialists recommend regular massage to boost a baby's health and well-being. Because holding and stroking your baby is a natural instinct, a daily massage can also help to bond your relationship, calm and soothe your child, and enhance a sense of security and love.

Light, slow strokes form the basis of a baby massage, providing comfort and allowing the infant to develop a sense of touch. There is no set pattern to the techniques, since every baby reacts differently; you can adjust the routine by judging the responses. Although some aromatherapy oils are safe for children, they should not be used on babies.

1 *Begin the massage with an all-over stroke, starting at the top of the head and gently running your fingertips down to the toes. Although some babies are more comfortable lying on either their backs or their stomachs, you can try turning your baby over and working on both sides of the body.*

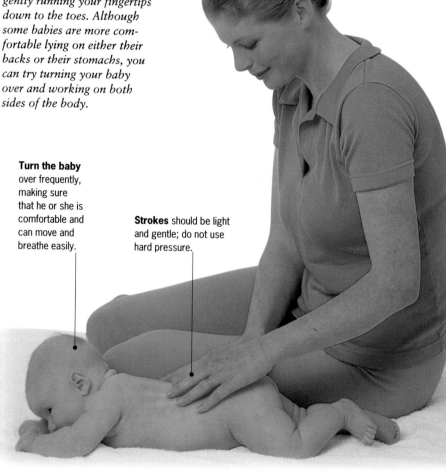

Turn the baby over frequently, making sure that he or she is comfortable and can move and breathe easily.

Strokes should be light and gentle; do not use hard pressure.

LIFESTYLE TIPS

▶ Warm baths improve blood circulation and provide gentle relaxation for babies and small children.

▶ Holding your baby often will promote feelings of security and love; a happy baby is more likely to be healthy.

▶ Babies like to have their limbs moved around, and it is good for their growth and flexibility. Try quickly bending and straightening the baby's arms and legs.

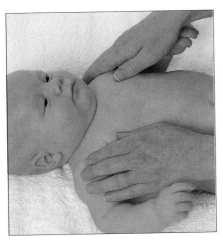

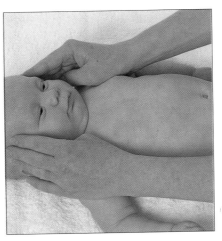

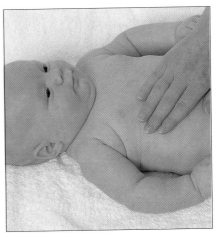

2 *With a little more force, stroke up the legs and over the stomach to the shoulders, then down the arms. Repeat as many times as you want.*

3 *Stroke from the top of the nose, around the temples, and down the sides of the face. Lightly stroke down from the eyes, around the mouth, and under the chin.*

4 *Run your fingertips clockwise around your baby's navel, increasing the size of the circles as you go and using more of your whole hand. This is good for stomach problems.*

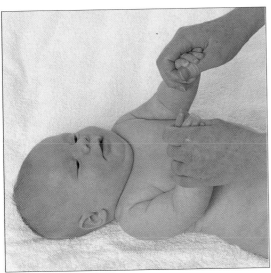

5 *Taking each of your baby's hands in yours, stretch the arms to their maximum length. Then bend them toward the body and straighten them again several times. This will increase flexibility and aid the development of the arm muscles.*

6 *Lift one leg and bend and stretch the knee three times. Take the leg through the full extent of its movement. Holding the foot, stroke up the leg to the abdomen. Repeat with the other leg. This improves the flexibility and mobility of the legs and enhances proper and strong development.*

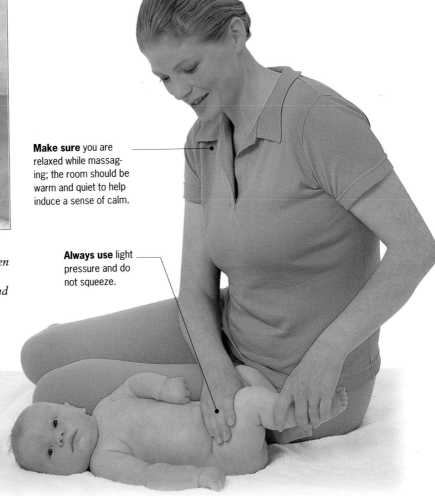

Make sure you are relaxed while massaging; the room should be warm and quiet to help induce a sense of calm.

Always use light pressure and do not squeeze.

Children can be massaged in the same way as babies, although they may not want to hold still for long, so it might be better to keep the session short. Making it part of a game will help them enjoy it and reduce the likelihood of boredom. The child doesn't need to undress and can be massaged wearing light clothing with no shoes.

Massage can do much to build a strong, positive relationship between parents and children, as well as between siblings and friends, thus increasing security.

You can also encourage your child to massage you. Most children love to touch and be touched, and you can make massage into a game while teaching them about the human body and how it works. Start off by teaching them simple stroking of the back and kneading of the shoulders. If the child is small (under five years old), you can ask him or her to walk up and down your back carefully. This will help ease any stresses and strains. (Make it clear, however, that your child should never practice this technique on friends.)

AROMATHERAPY

It is safe to use aromatherapy oils on children in weak dilutions (half the strength that an adult would normally use). Take particular care with oils known to cause problems for sensitive skin.

▶ *Chamomile and/or lavender for calming*

▶ *Orange and/or chamomile for colic*

▶ *Sandalwood and/or lavender for insomnia*

▶ *Tea tree and/or eucalyptus for coughs and colds*

Before using essential oils for massage, please read the information on safety and general use given on pages 152–156.

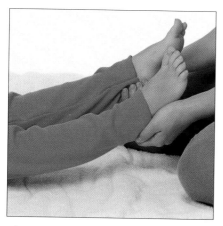

1 *Start by holding onto the feet and giving the legs a good shake. Then alternately bend each leg to its full extent. Repeat several times.*

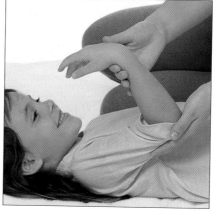

2 *Take one hand and shake the arm, then bend the wrist, elbow, and shoulder to their full extent. Repeat with the other arm.*

4 *Finish off by gently stroking the scalp through the hair. Make sure that you use long, even strokes and cover all of the head area.*

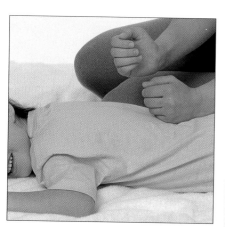

3 *Gently pummel up the back with your hands lightly clenched and parallel to each other. Ask the child to say "AAAHH" loudly as you do it. This will aid breathing and loosen any phlegm in the chest and throat.*

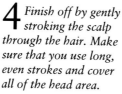

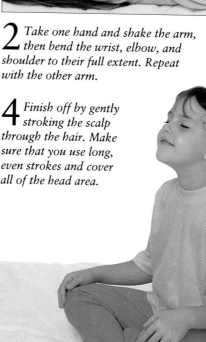

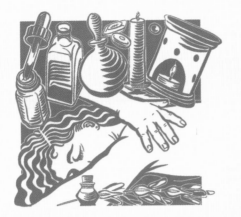

CHAPTER 6

HEAL
YOURSELF
WITH TOUCH

*Everyone can enjoy the pleasures and healing
qualities of touch. Basic massage techniques are
easy to learn and come naturally to most people.
Massaging your partner, family members, or
friends can bring you closer and cement your
relationships. Alternatively, a quiet self-massage
will release tension in your muscles and give you
some time by yourself to relax and unwind.*

HOME MASSAGE

Massage can be a wonderful way to become more intimate with a special friend or partner. With a little planning, you can turn your home into a sanctuary for healing and relaxation.

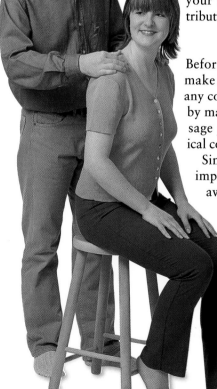

Most people have massage because they enjoy the feel of it and the relaxation it brings. But massage is not just an enjoyable experience that lasts for the duration of the session. It can make a general contribution to good health and happiness without any adverse side effects. Home massage costs nothing in monetary terms but pays big dividends in many other ways. Touch conveys to the receiver a feeling of being cared for, and in fact, a good massage can be given only by someone who cares. Time devoted to sharing massage becomes special time, the one thing that is often lacking in our modern way of life.

Even without a partner, you can use massage on your own body to achieve good effects. Through self-massage you can stimulate blood flow, relieve muscle tension, improve lymph drainage, and increase your energy, all of which greatly contribute to good health and well-being.

SAFETY ISSUES

Before massaging someone, you must make sure that he or she doesn't have any condition that could be made worse by massage. It is often harmful to massage people who have any of the medical conditions listed on page 43.

Since the skin bears the immediate impact of a massage, you should be aware of any allergic conditions that could be aggravated by pressure, rubbing, or the active ingredients in essential oils. It is also not recommended to have massage immediately following a heavy meal. Although cancer does not contraindicate all forms of touch therapy, a patient should consult his doctor beforehand, giving full details of the kind of massage planned. Heart conditions and excessively high blood pressure should be regarded in the same way. People who have osteoporosis can receive light soft-tissue massage but no joint manipulations. Anyone suffering from epilepsy is advised to avoid all but the very lightest massage.

There are some other things to consider before giving a massage. You should not give one if you are under the influence of alcohol or drugs. It is also inadvisable to massage another person if you have an infectious skin condition, a fever, or are suffering from a cold or the flu.

Attention to posture is vital if you give frequent massages. Keep your back upright and use your entire body weight, not just your hands and arms, to create deeper pressure. Change positions often, and stop if you feel any pain or discomfort yourself. This is more likely to happen when you are using manipulative massage techniques.

MASSAGE EQUIPMENT

At the most basic level, a pair of hands and a little space are the only requirements for a massage, although having a comfortable and relaxing setting will almost certainly increase the pleasure. Aromatherapy oils can also be used to enhance massage.

There are stores that specialize in massage and touch therapy equipment, often stocking a range of aromatherapy essential oils as well. However, a homemade alternative is sometimes just as good as purchased equipment—sometimes better—and usually a great deal less expensive.

Massage couches

Before investing in a massage couch, try the floor. You need only a couple of thick blankets or an exercise mat to provide a padded surface. However, if you find it difficult to

MASSAGE CLASSES

Joining a massage class is a good way to learn basic techniques or improve your skills before working on friends and family members, and at the same time you can enjoy other students practicing on you. You don't need a partner to join a class; in fact, it provides an ideal opportunity for finding a massage partner. If you can't find a massage school in your area, see if a local college or community center would be willing to offer classes. Or ask a massage institute if their practitioners also give training.

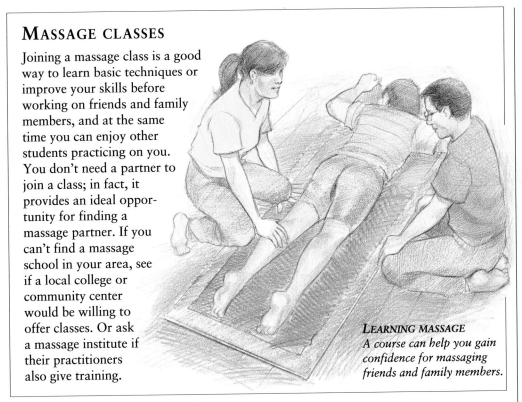

LEARNING MASSAGE
A course can help you gain confidence for massaging friends and family members.

give a massage in the kneeling position, the best alternative is to find a proper massage couch. There are many kinds available. Be sure the height is adjustable, and if possible, buy a couch with a face hole. This keeps the recipient's neck in a relaxed position during the massage. Tables and beds do not generally make good alternatives but will do in a pinch. If you are using a bed, it should have a very firm base and mattress. On a table, use blankets for padding.

Towels

If you are using oil, you will need a large towel to protect the massage couch, bed, or blankets plus additional ones with which to drape the recipient during the session. It is important to have a good supply of towels of varying sizes on hand, because it is awkward to interrupt a massage should you need more of them.

There are no particular towels that are better for massage, but fresh and clean ones in solid colors rather than busy patterns are preferable. Professionals usually prefer large, soft, white towels, which they keep warm and replace frequently.

Loofahs, brushes, and rollers

There is a large variety of items available at many pharmacies and stores that stock mas-sage equipment. Loofahs and other natural sponges and skin brushes can be used to remove dead cells, nourishing and cleaning the skin thoroughly. Rollers and massage balls, which are fun and easy to use, can be rolled against the skin to produce a kneading effect. These items are not necessary for a good massage, however, and most professional masseurs do not use them.

MASSAGING A PARTNER

Massage can be an enjoyable pastime for couples, encouraging relaxation and good health. Many couples see it as a special time when they can enjoy each other's company and intimacy—an expression of their partnership and affection. Couples often use this time alone to reestablish closeness and talk

DID YOU KNOW?

Different parts of the body respond to touch in specific ways. The skin of the face is most sensitive to being touched, whereas the skin on the hands is most sensitive to feeling other things. The sense of touch also varies from one person to another; characteristically, women are more sensitive both to being touched and to touching than men are.

TIPS FOR THE MASSEUR

The person giving a massage should bear in mind these guidelines:

▶ *Wear something comfortable that allows free movement.*

▶ *Take off all jewelry and watches.*

▶ *Tie your hair back if it is long or likely to distract you.*

▶ *Don't wear any strong perfume, especially if you are using aromatherapy oils.*

▶ *Make sure that you are relaxed; take a few deep breaths before you begin.*

▶ *Maintain good posture and make sure that you don't tense your muscles, because this will disturb your natural rhythm.*

▶ *Take your time, flowing from one movement into another.*

▶ *Make sure that you won't be interrupted. Take the phone off the hook and ask others not to disturb you.*

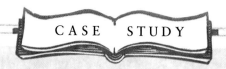
A Problem with Sex

Sexual problems can be embarrassing and awkward, making it easy to put them to the back of your mind and busy yourself with other things. However, problems with sex can seriously disrupt a good relationship, breaking down communication between two people and causing lingering resentment and mistrust. Good sexual relations can be restored with the help of massage techniques.

Tom is a busy professional in his early forties. He has been married to Kay for 16 years, but their marriage is breaking down and they no longer enjoy a good sex life. Tom is aware that sex is still important to him, although he has become progressively more embarrassed about his sexual performance. He has distanced himself from Kay because he feels that he cannot discuss his problems, and he has thrown himself into his work to compensate. Also, Tom is spending most evenings out with his friends drinking. The couple has sought the advice of a marriage counselor, who suggests that their relationship would improve if they worked through their sexual problems with the help of a sex therapist.

WHAT SHOULD TOM DO?

Tom and Kay should go to a sex therapist, who will first ask them about their sexual histories and problems. The therapist will consider whether Tom needs to have a medical checkup to make sure that his body is functioning properly and determine if treatment is necessary. The therapist will help Tom to accept and understand his problems and work them out rather than ignoring them. Tom and Kay both may be asked to follow a course of sensate focus (see page 126), a home massage program that promotes physical communication, understanding, and acceptance. In their case, this would put particular emphasis on Tom's problems with sexual performance.

Action Plan

LIFESTYLE
Make time to focus on developing intimacy with Kay. Although friends and career are important, the relationship must come first.

SEX LIFE
Although it may be difficult, talk to Kay about problems with sex: bringing difficulties into the open is the first step to understanding and resolving them.

STRESS
Undertake a course of massage to relieve stress, become more relaxed, and improve confidence and self-image.

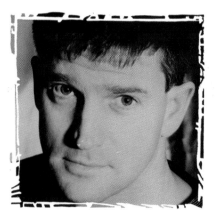

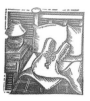

LIFESTYLE
A busy and over-active lifestyle can be a way of excusing yourself from facing problems in your personal life.

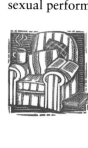

SEX LIFE
If you and your partner are not open and communicative about sexual problems and anxieties, your sex life can suffer and may break down completely.

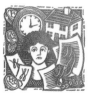

STRESS
Having doubts about your own self-image can have a negative effect on your sex life.

HOW THINGS TURNED OUT FOR TOM

The sex therapist helped Tom understand his sexual problems, and eventually his self-esteem was restored, and confidence in his sexual ability returned. Tom and Kay followed the course of sensate focus and found that massage enabled them to relax and feel comfortable with their own bodies. Through massage they have gotten to know each other again, communication between them has improved, and they have started to regain a close and intimate relationship.

about their relationship, any problems, or plans they have for the future.

Massage can also be good for relationship problems. Marriage counselors often advise couples who are having problems to touch each other more, particularly by hugging and massaging. Through massage, couples can get to know each other's bodies better and understand where touch is well received. It can also provide invaluable time alone with each other, restoring a sense of intimacy in the relationship.

Sex problems can be mitigated by massage (see page 126). It can enable a person to feel more comfortable with his or her body, get used to and enjoy being touched, and learn to relax more readily.

MASSAGING A FRIEND

Massaging a friend can be a wonderful way to become closer to that person. If you are new friends, possibly two people who have met in massage class, you may find that you build up trust as you practice techniques.

The best massages are those that do not involve sexual actions or motives. However, in a society in which touch and nudity are readily connected with sexual intimacy, problems and misunderstandings can arise in a massage situation. Whether you are massaging a partner or a friend, it is important that both of you be comfortable and feel no obligation to do anything that you don't want to. Building up a good massage relationship can be awkward at first. To avoid any misunderstandings, explain fully what you intend to do.

Clothing

Usually the person being massaged wears nothing or only underwear, and towels are used to cover the parts of the body that are not being massaged. For Eastern massage techniques, loose cotton clothing is best, worn without restrictive underwear.

Many people feel uncomfortable if they are not wearing clothes because society's strict codes have, since the Victorian era, associated nudity with sexual intimacy. Since most massages are easier and more enjoyable without clothing, it is important to separate massage from sexual intimacy and reevaluate your attitude toward nudity. If you feel comfortable and relaxed with it, then you will convey your confidence to your massage partner.

Alternatively, you can try massage therapies that do not require you to take off your clothing. These include Oriental massages such as Tuina and shiatsu and massages that focus on the feet or the head.

SELF-MASSAGE

Self-massage gives you an opportunity to concentrate on yourself and think about your life, trying to see problems in perspective and working out practical solutions. It can also be deeply relaxing, calming, and rejuvenating, especially if you can imagine yourself on a warm golden beach or in another soothing place at the same time.

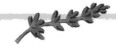

CUTICLE CREAM

This is an excellent cream for conditioning your nails and keeping your hands in good shape. The tea tree oil is a disinfectant that will also help prevent common fungal infections of the nails.

10 g (⅓ oz) beeswax pieces
60 ml (4 tbsp) almond oil

5 drops lavender essential oil
10 drops tea tree essential oil

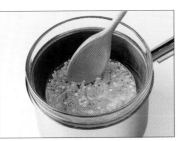

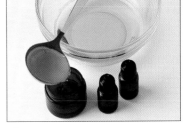

1 *Gently heat the beeswax and almond oil in a heatproof bowl over a pan of simmering water. When the beeswax has melted, remove from the heat and stir.*

2 *Stir in the essential oils. Pour the mixture into a screw-top jar and allow it to cool, then close the jar firmly.*

3 *Trim and file your nails. Massage a small amount of cuticle cream into each nail and gently push the cuticles back with a cuticle stick. Wipe off any excess cuticle cream. You can apply this cream daily to soften the cuticles or use it whenever you do a full-hand manicure.*

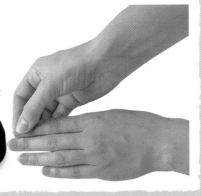

SETTING THE SCENE

The place you choose for a massage should have a welcoming ambience and, above all, be private. It should be a space separated from everyday life to allow peaceful relaxation.

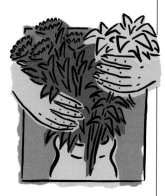

IMPROVING YOUR TOUCH

Feeling, picking, and arranging flowers can help you improve your sense of touch, as well as your sense of smell. Feel the textures of petals, leaves, and stems. How do they compare? Rub them between your fingers. What scents do they emit?

Home massage can be a highly enjoyable and relaxing experience, and its pleasure can be enhanced by creating an atmosphere conducive to relaxation and contemplation. This is especially important if you or your partner find it difficult to relax, are particularly stressed, or feel in any way shy toward each other. There are many ways in which you can help to make the mood feel right.

MAKING TIME

Probably one of the most important considerations is making time for a massage when you won't be interrupted by others. About one hour is needed for two people to massage each other and about 30 minutes for a full self-massage. Try to plan a massage in advance, establishing the exact time that it will start and finish, so that you can work it into the rest of your day. Stating a specific starting time will allow you to enter the mood straight away, leaving behind your other concerns.

FENG SHUI

If you are interested in Oriental massage, you might want to use Feng Shui to enhance your room and furnishings. This is the traditional Chinese art of balancing energy flows in your surroundings in order to improve your well-being. It advises on shapes, colors, and materials for a room's elements and tells how to position them to enhance the flow of universal energy, or qi. According to Feng Shui, the best materials for massage would be soft-edged and made of natural fibers in soft or natural colors.

If you want to have a shorter self-massage a few times a week or even every day, try to get into a routine. It might be easy, for example, to put aside 10 minutes every evening after a warm bath to unwind and rub out the day's stresses.

MAKING SPACE

Although massage can be done virtually anywhere, the best place is a quiet and uncluttered room where you can count on complete privacy. It is important that both you and your partner feel at ease, so try to find a familiar place where you will be comfortable and can avoid being disturbed. Some people find it beneficial to lock the door, giving them the knowledge that they are in a secure space.

ROOM FURNISHINGS

An uncluttered room with plenty of space around the massage area is best because it allows for ease of movement. The fewer the distractions the better, so make sure that attention-drawing objects are covered or put away. Soft, warm colors will induce relaxation and the release of stress. Avoid using hard-edged furniture and create a comfortable feeling with soft cushions and towels.

Subdued lighting will also enable you to relax and take your mind away from your everyday worries. This is especially helpful if the person being massaged feels shy, even wearing clothes. Candles produce a warm, moving light, which can greatly enhance the atmosphere. An open fire produces a flickering glow, which throws a gentle light into a room, although additional dim lights may also be needed.

It is important to warm up the room before you start a massage, because cold skin will not readily absorb oils and will not be supple. Ideally, the room temperature should be a comfortable 24°C (75°F).

MUSIC

The relaxing effects of certain kinds of music are well known, and soft music can be a perfect accompaniment for massage. Because people have their own tastes in relaxing music, check with your partner beforehand so that you can choose something that will please both of you. Play it softly in the background. For the person giving the massage, soft music can aid in keeping the rhythm and centering the mind.

CLOTHING

If you are wearing clothes, they should be loose, light, and preferably made from cotton. Shoes must not be worn, and it will create a better mood if you leave them outside. Do not wear any tight underwear because it will directly affect the massage strokes. Both you and your partner should remove all jewelry before you start.

When no clothes are to be worn, towels can be used to cover the areas not being massaged. This will help keep the skin warm as well as respect the modesty of the person being massaged.

SCENT

Releasing scents with an aromatherapy burner, a dish set above a candle, will help to complete the perfect massage ambience. Choose a relaxing essential oil such as chamomile or lavender and pour a few drops with a little water into the burner. Scented candles can also be effective. These are usually available in card and gift shops.

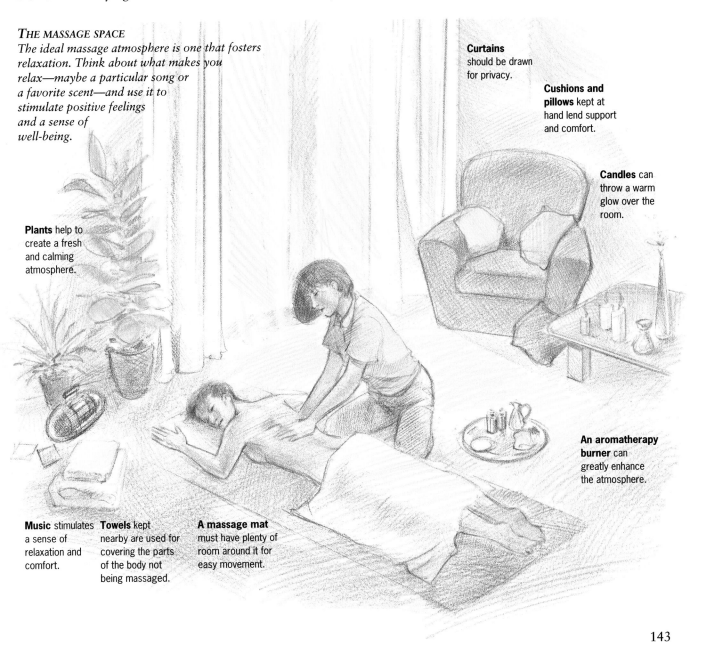

THE MASSAGE SPACE
The ideal massage atmosphere is one that fosters relaxation. Think about what makes you relax—maybe a particular song or a favorite scent—and use it to stimulate positive feelings and a sense of well-being.

Curtains should be drawn for privacy.

Cushions and pillows kept at hand lend support and comfort.

Candles can throw a warm glow over the room.

Plants help to create a fresh and calming atmosphere.

An aromatherapy burner can greatly enhance the atmosphere.

Music stimulates a sense of relaxation and comfort.

Towels kept nearby are used for covering the parts of the body not being massaged.

A massage mat must have plenty of room around it for easy movement.

Tuina Body Massage

Tuina aims to rebalance the body's energy through massage and stimulation of the acupressure points. The techniques used here are described in Swedish Massage Strokes (pages 44–47) and in Eastern Massage Techniques (pages 57–60).

Tuina massage is a traditional Chinese system of hands-on healing that involves soft-tissue techniques and manipulations. It achieves its remarkable results by working on the energy channels, or meridians, and their acupressure points. This guide to Tuina includes only a few of the many techniques used by a traditional Chinese doctor. Though simple, these do produce very positive results, helping to relieve stress and making you feel revitalized and refreshed. The person being massaged will be clothed throughout except for shoes. Cotton sweatpants and a T-shirt are ideal. For the neck and shoulder massage, a chair or stool is required. Tuina is easy to learn and can be done at home with your friends and family.

THE NECK

For a neck and shoulder massage, a firm chair or stool is required. Make sure that the recipient is relaxed by having her practice deep breathing before you start (see page 38).

1 *With a kneading action, squeeze the neck on both sides of the spine, using the thumb and fingers of your right hand. Keep your fingers straight and apply their fleshy pads when squeezing. As the recipient becomes used to the pressure, you can increase it progressively. Change hands frequently and support the forehead with the hand that is not squeezing.*

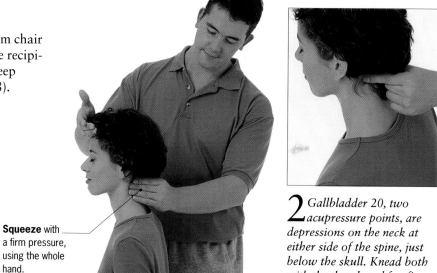

Squeeze with a firm pressure, using the whole hand.

BENEFITS

Treating a person once or twice a week will keep neck pain at bay. Gallbladder 20 is a key point for relieving headaches and aching eyes. Gallbladder 21 affects neck and shoulder pains and muscle stiffness.

2 *Gallbladder 20, two acupressure points, are depressions on the neck at either side of the spine, just below the skull. Knead both with the thumb and forefinger.*

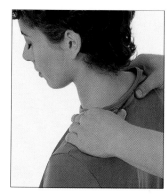

3 *Gallbladder 21 is midway between two points: the spine at the base of the neck and the back corner of the shoulder bone.*

THE SHOULDERS

The shoulders harbor much of the body's stress and related tension. A Tuina session on the shoulders can enhance relaxation and help overcome tension headaches and other problems associated with stress and tension buildup.

1 *Stand behind the recipient and start the massage with a few light presses on top of the shoulders, using both hands. Progressively change the pressing action into a squeezing one, squeezing with both hands in unison.*

Make sure that the recipient is sitting upright with a good posture.

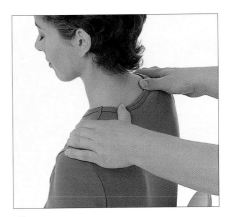

2 *Gradually change from using the heels of the palms to the full length of the thumbs. Knead deeply with them, starting on either side of the spine and moving out toward the shoulders.*

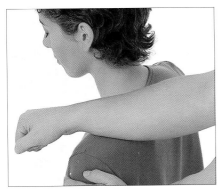

3 *Place the underside of your right forearm over the left shoulder of the recipient, in the crease between the shoulder and neck, and lean gently into the body. Repeat on the other side.*

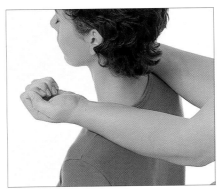

4 *Palms facing upward, place both of your forearms on the shoulders of the recipient at the same time. Gently lean on the shoulders, feeling for tension to ease from the shoulder area.*

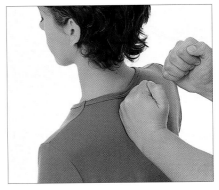

5 *Steadily pummel the upper back and shoulders with the outer edges of lightly clenched, or half-open, fists. Make sure that you ask the recipient to tell you if you are using too much pressure.*

THE ARMS

Stresses in our daily lives often cause tension to build up in the arms. This is then transmitted to the shoulders, causing tension, tiredness, and pain. All types of massage can be beneficial to the arms, but particularly Tuina, because the arms carry six major meridians and working on these will revitalize the energy flow throughout the system. The person being massaged remains seated throughout the routine.

1 Grasp the recipient's hand in both of yours, with your thumbs lying side by side along the top of the wrist. Lean back slightly to produce a light pull on the arm and shake it with fast up-and-down movements at least 10 times. Repeat with the other arm.

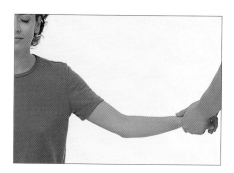

2 Standing behind the shoulder, grasp the recipient's wrist, lean her arm on your thigh, and with your other hand, squeeze up and down the outside of the arm with a slight lifting action. Holding the arm a little higher, turn it over and squeeze up and down the inside, using a firm grip around the upper arm.

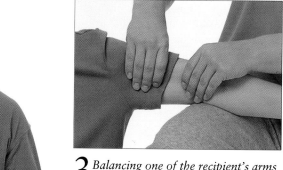

3 Balancing one of the recipient's arms on your thigh, knead thoroughly up the arm with both hands together. Repeat on the other arm.

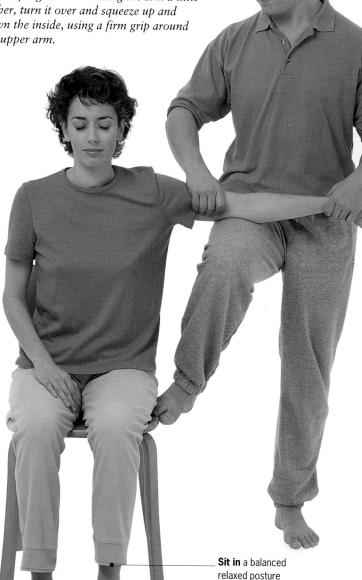

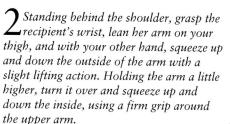

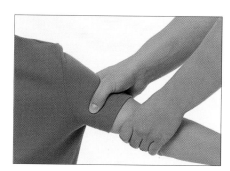

4 Taking an arm firmly in both hands, use a twisting movement to loosen the soft tissues and muscles. Work your way down the arm. Repeat with other arm.

Sit in a balanced relaxed posture throughout the session.

BENEFITS

Tuina places strong emphasis on massaging the arms because six meridians pass through them. Shaking is particularly beneficial because it stimulates and improves circulation, which in turn eases joint pain and stimulates the flow of energy.

THE BACK AND BUTTOCKS

It is amazing how much tension can be stored in the back and buttocks, but most Western massage sequences pay scant attention to the buttocks area. This very simple massage can relieve sciatica and lower back pain and ease tension. It also restores proper energy flow along the important Bladder meridian.

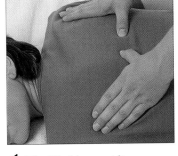

1 *The Bladder meridian runs two finger widths from either side of the spine. Use thumb pressure all the way down.*

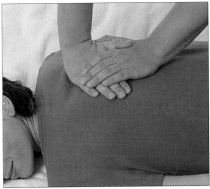

2 *Cross the fingers of one hand over those of the other and place the heels of both palms on the muscled area to the left of the spine just below the neck. Use circular movements and increase the pressure by leaning in with your body weight. Repeat on the other side.*

3 *Place both hands flat across the back with your thumbs together, then put pressure onto the whole spine area. This will relieve energy blocks in the Bladder meridian.*

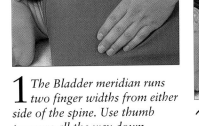

Pressure in this massage should come from the shoulders.

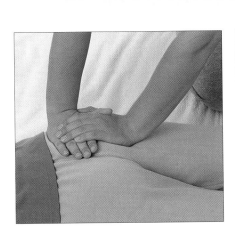

4 *On the right side facing the buttocks, place one hand on top of the other and knead deeply, using the heels of your hands. Repeat on the other side.*

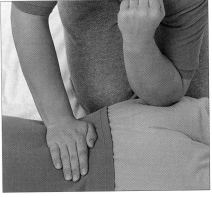

5 *Using your elbow, push firmly into the whole buttock area, using small circular movements. However, do not apply too much pressure.*

BENEFITS

A good spine massage benefits the body for many reasons, not least through stimulating the Bladder meridian, which runs alongside it. The massage described above is powerful. It will relieve back pain of all kinds, migraines and other headaches, stress, depression, and insomnia. Without detailed knowledge of the acupressure points, however, you cannot treat specific conditions.

THE LEGS

Some of the most powerful parts of the meridian system run down the legs, and massage can help to ease pains and tensions. Stomach 36 is an important acupressure point and is used to boost the immune system and treat stomach problems.

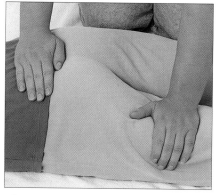

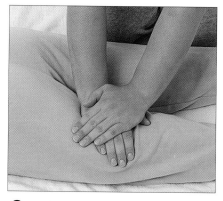

1 *Place your hand on the back of the thigh and squeeze all the way down the leg to the ankle. Squeeze lightly at first, using a slight lifting action on the tissues that you grasp. Repeat, lifting your hand back up to the thigh.*

2 *With one hand over the other, place large circular pressure firmly all the way down the leg. The pressure should come from the body weight of the masseur. Move to the other side and repeat steps 1 and 2 on the other leg.*

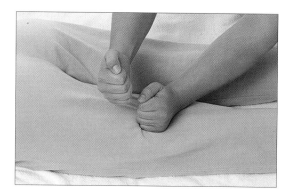

3 *With your fists lightly clasped, pummel gently down each leg. You can pummel the thigh more deeply than the calf. Do not pummel behind the knee or the ankle, as this may cause joint damage.*

BENEFITS

This leg massage aims to improve the energy flow in the six meridians that run down each leg. It can help to relieve back pain, sciatica, and sports injuries to the hamstring, as well as ease emotional strains.

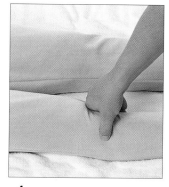

4 *Stomach 36 lies four finger widths beneath the kneecap and one finger width away from the outside of the shinbone. Press with the thumb for 2 minutes.*

5 *Repeat the squeezing, kneading and pummeling techniques of steps 1, 2, and 3 on the front of the thigh.*

THE HANDS

The hands are particularly sensitive parts of the body, being able to touch and feel pressure easily. An important acupressure point, Large Intestine 4, can stimulate the immune system and treat headaches and migraine, toothache and anxiety.

BENEFITS

The acupressure point Large Intestine 4 can be used to stimulate the immune system and balance the energies in the head and face. It can also treat stress disorders, confusion, and insomnia, and can boost general well-being. It must not be used if you are pregnant.

THE FEET

Feet are very sensitive and respond to many of our inner feelings and emotions. Witness the way people are ticklish or jump when you touch their feet. Opening the meridians on the feet can be greatly relieving, restoring balance and a sense of groundedness, solidity, and well-being.

BENEFITS

Pummeling makes the tissues of the feet receptive to energy flow and opens the meridians to allow a balanced stream of energy. Stimulating the acupressure point Kidney 1 brings energy down the body to produce a feeling of being grounded and calm. It can also relieve insomnia and confusion.

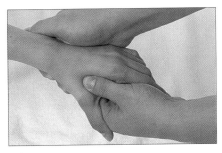

1 *Large Intestine 4 can be found on the web between the thumb and index finger, where you feel the bones on either side. Knead this point deeply for 1 minute with your thumb.*

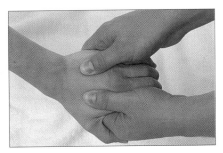

2 *Use the pad of your thumb to knead with small circular movements all the tendons along the back of the recipient's hand. Also gently knead the joints of each finger in turn.*

CAUTION

Large Intestine 4 is a very powerful acupressure point and must not be used during pregnancy, as it can cause miscarriage.

1 *Lift the foot in one hand and pummel the sole with the other. Use firmer pressure on the heel.*

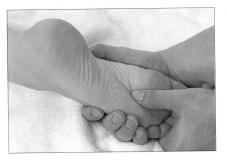

2 *Press and knead the acupressure point Kidney 1. This is a depression in the center of the sole, two-thirds up the foot from the heel.*

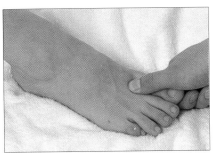

3 *Use thumb pressure to push into the entire foot, top and bottom. Start at the edge of the foot and then work inward, covering the entire area.*

Tuina Self-Massage

Set aside 10 minutes every day or a few times a week to get in touch with your body. Some of the methods used are described in Swedish Massage Strokes (pages 44–47) and in Eastern Massage Techniques (pages 57–60).

THE HEAD

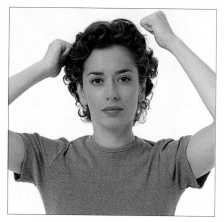

With your back straight, raise your arms up on both sides and gently pummel your head all over.

THE ARMS

1 *Start by shaking both wrists until they flop around loosely. Clench your right fist lightly and use the bent fingers to pummel gently up the outside of your left arm.*

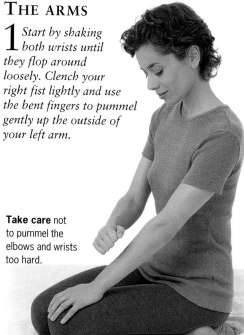

Take care not to pummel the elbows and wrists too hard.

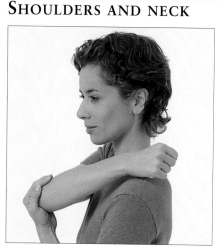

2 *When you reach the shoulder, turn your left arm so that the palm faces upward and pummel down the inside. Repeat this about 10 times, increasing the pressure as you get used to the feel of it. Now do the other arm.*

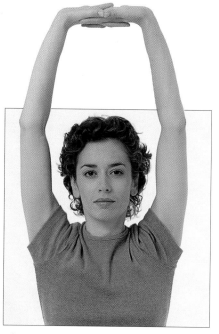

1 *Stretch the muscles and joints in your shoulders by clasping your hands together above your head and pulling straight up. This releases energy blocks.*

SHOULDERS AND NECK

2 *Supporting your elbow, use the pummeling technique along the top of the shoulders. Start with the right hand pummeling the left shoulder.*

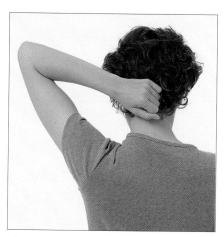

3 *Pummel up the back of the neck, taking care not to use too much force. The sides of the neck particularly will benefit from pummeling.*

THE CHEST

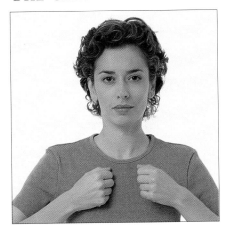

Clench your hands loosely and place them on either side of your chest, ready for pummeling. Breathe out as much as you can and then take a very deep breath. Now start pummeling and breathe out slowly at the same time, making a steady "AAAAHH" sound until you run out of breath. Repeat several times. This moves the lung energies and boosts the immune system.

THE LEGS

1 *Bend forward, allowing your hands to hang loosely. Feel the muscles stretching in the back of your legs and your shoulders. This helps loosen the meridians.*

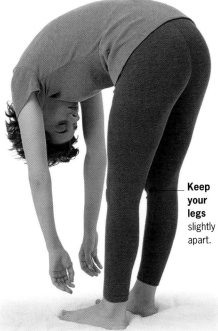

Keep your legs slightly apart.

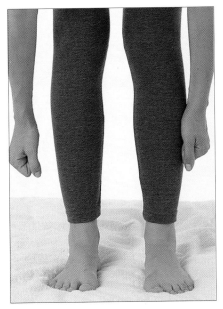

2 *Pummel alternately down the outside of both legs to the ankles and up the insides of the legs. Repeat several times. This stimulates energy flow in the six meridians of the legs.*

THE BACK AND BUTTOCKS

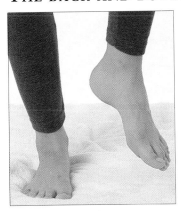

1 *Stand on one foot and shake the other to loosen the ankle and assist energy flow in the leg meridians. Now shake the other foot in the same way.*

2 *Pummel alternately down the back and onto the buttocks and then return up to the starting point, pummeling as you go. Repeat the complete cycle several times. If you have recently suffered lower back pain, do this carefully.*

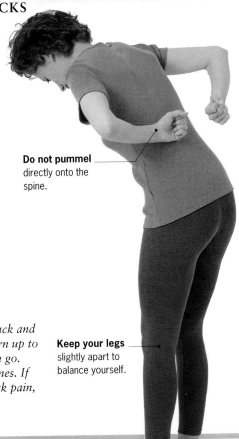

Do not pummel directly onto the spine.

Keep your legs slightly apart to balance yourself.

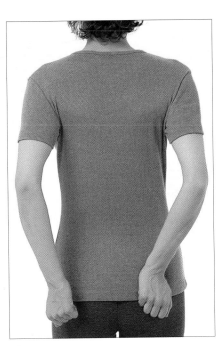

3 *The buttocks area requires harder pressure than the back and must be pummeled all over. This stimulates the kidneys and helps relieve back pain.*

AROMATHERAPY

The combination of Swedish massage with aromatherapy massage oils has become popular for its therapeutic impact, providing both physical and emotional relief and relaxation.

USING ESSENTIAL OILS SAFELY

Read this section carefully before using essential oils.

► *Never take essential oils internally.*

► *Do not be tempted to add more essential oil than directed, as only a few drops will have a powerful effect.*

► *Do a skin test 48 hours before using an oil if you have sensitive skin.*

► *Check with a doctor first if you are pregnant, epileptic, or suffering from any serious illness.*

► *If you will be going out in the sun, do not use any oil that is photo-toxic, that is, for which a stated safety precaution is "Avoid exposure to ultraviolet light" (see pages 154–155).*

There is no doubt that essential oils have healing qualities and a general uplifting effect. It is believed that when inhaled, the healing properties of the oils are absorbed through the lungs into the bloodstream. When applied as part of massage, they are absorbed through the skin.

Although the use of essential oils was an ancient and traditional art, their medicinal qualities were rediscovered in modern times by René Gattefossé, a French chemist working in his family perfumery in the early 20th century. When he burned himself severely in a laboratory accident, he found that lavender oil relieved the pain. A French army physician carried out further research on essential oils during World War II, and Marguerite Maury, an Austrian biochemist, extended the uses of oils by creating the concept of the individual prescription. By the 1970s they had become well known as healing and massage tools.

ESSENTIAL OILS
The essential oils used in aromatherapy are chemically complex. Extracted from the original plant sources by a process of steam distillation, or expression, they are highly concentrated liquids which should never be applied undiluted onto the skin and should always be used with caution. There are more than 300 different essential oils, each with its own particular healing properties. A list of some of the more common ones and their uses can be found on pages 154–155.

NOTES
In perfumery, essential oils are classified as corresponding to a "note," which describes their dynamic in the perfume. The heavier oils, which have slower evaporation rates, are the base notes; they generally last the longest. The middle notes are believed to balance a blend. The top notes are the oils, like lemon, that can be smelled first but evaporate quickly.

CARRIER OR BASE OILS
Carrier, or base, oils are used in massage to help the movements of the hands smoother over the body and to moisturize the skin of the recipient. They are usually cold-pressed vegetable oils, which can be very beneficial

continued on page 156

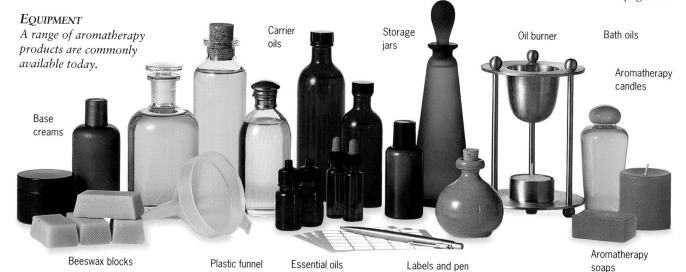

EQUIPMENT
A range of aromatherapy products are commonly available today.

Carrier oils

Storage jars

Oil burner

Bath oils

Aromatherapy candles

Base creams

Beeswax blocks

Plastic funnel

Essential oils

Labels and pen

Aromatherapy soaps

Massage Oil

You can blend oils at home to create your own personal massage oil for enhancing your mood and treating any ailments you might have. Learning about the qualities of different oils and what they can do for you can be enjoyable and rewarding.

To calculate how many drops of an essential oil can be added to a massage oil, start with the amount—in milliliters—of the base, or carrier, oil to be used, then divide this amount by 2. For example, 20 ml (about 4 teaspoons) is usually enough carrier oil for a full-body massage, so to this you would add 10 drops of one or more essential oils.

Most aromatherapy suppliers now also stock base creams and lotions that are free from any perfume or other additives. With these you can create your own aromatherapy moisturizers and body lotions with the addition of essential oils. Using the same guidelines as for the base oil, divide the amount of base cream in milliliters by 2 to determine the amount of essential oil to add. For example, 50 ml of cream will take 25 drops of essential oil.

Essential oils can also be used in compresses. Pour 6 drops of oil into a large bowl of hot water, then place a facecloth on the water's surface to collect the film of oil. Wring it out and place it on your forehead, feet, or other problem area, for 10 to 20 minutes, resoaking the cloth as it cools.

Inhalations can be very effective at relieving respiratory problems. Stir 2 to 6 drops of essential oil into a large bowl of boiling water and place a towel over it. Allow it to cool slightly, then lean your head over the bowl, covering your head with the towel.

STORING OILS
Both essential oils and massage blends should be kept in dark glass bottles in a cool, dry environment. Make sure that you label them clearly.

MAKING AN INDIVIDUAL MASSAGE OIL

Mixing your own massage oil is easy and allows you to create the right blend for you. Check the table on pages 154–155 to find out which of the essential oils will provide the best results for your individual needs. Read the warnings carefully and do not exceed the recommended amount; it could cause an allergic reaction or drowsiness.

SPECIAL BLENDS

By blending your own essential oils, you can create special aromas and obtain all the healing qualities that meet your specific requirements. Below are three examples of popular mixes to start you off. Remember, you should never exceed the recommended amounts.

STRESS-RELIEVING MASSAGE OIL
To 20 ml almond oil, add
3 drops neroli
4 drops lavender
3 drops bergamot

LUXURIOUSLY UPLIFTING MASSAGE OIL
To 20 ml almond oil, add
2 drops patchouli
4 drops rose
4 drops bergamot

OIL FOR ACHES AND PAINS
To 20 ml almond oil, add
5 drops frankincense
3 drops lavender
2 drops rosemary

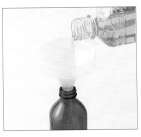

1 *Once you have decided on a mixture, pour 20 ml of carrier oil into a jar or bottle that closes firmly. Using a funnel prevents spillage.*

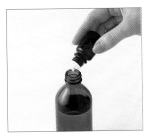

2 *Add no more than 10 drops in total of essential oils. Three oils are usually plenty for a good massage oil mix.*

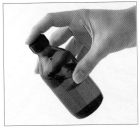

3 *Screw the top on and shake vigorously. Pour some onto the palm of one hand and rub your palms together to warm it before applying it to the body.*

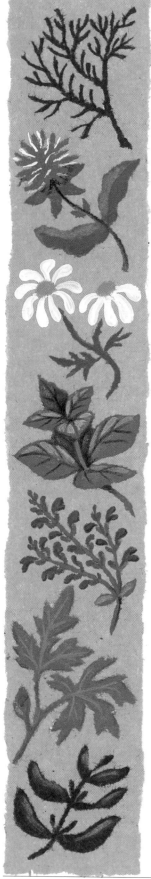

ESSENTIAL OILS

An essential oil is broadly described as having a stimulating, sedating, uplifting or regulating quality, although every oil within these groups will also possess other qualities. The "note" of an oil can be top, middle or base. It will be base if it is a slow evaporating oil, and top if the scent fades quickly. A good blend will contain a mixture of top, middle, and base notes. Chapter 5 gives details of aromatherapy massage and recommended oils for certain conditions.

ESSENTIAL OIL	PROBLEMS TREATED	EMOTIONS TREATED	SAFETY PRECAUTIONS	NOTE
BASIL (stimulant)	Insect repellent, aches and pains, headaches lethargy, tiredness	Anxiety, depression, fatigue, insomnia	Avoid if pregnant or if you have sensitive skin.	Top
BENZOIN (sedating)	Arthritis, chapped and inflamed skin, colic, coughs, colds, flu	Anxiety, depression, loneliness, stress	Test first if you have sensitive skin.	Base
BERGAMOT (uplifting)	Cold sores, eczema, psoriasis, immune deficiency, infections, loss of appetite	Depression, stress-related problems, premenstrual syndrome	Avoid exposure to ultraviolet light.	Top
CHAMOMILE (sedating)	Chilblains, eczema, inflammation, aches, rheumatoid arthritis	Anger, irritability, insomnia, premenstrual syndrome	There are no specific safety precautions.	Middle
CLARY SAGE (uplifting)	Menstrual pain, muscle spasms and cramps, sore throat, childbirth problems	Anxiety, lack of sex drive, depression, tension-related disorders, premenstrual syndrome	Avoid if pregnant or if you are taking the contraceptive pill. Do not use with alcohol.	Middle
CLOVE (BUD) (uplifting)	Arthritis, rheumatic pains, digestive disorders, cystitis	Nervous exhaustion, nerves, panic	Avoid if you have sensitive skin.	Middle
CYPRESS (sedating)	Asthma, colds, heavy periods, cellulitis, oily and problem skin	Tension, stress, hyperactivity	Avoid if pregnant or if you have sensitive skin.	Middle
EUCALYPTUS (stimulant)	Bronchitis, coughs, colds, congestion, breathing difficulties, rheumatic pain, throat infections	Feelings of imbalance, lack of energy, tiredness	Avoid or test first if you have sensitive skin.	Top
FENNEL (stimulant)	Bloating, gas, cellulitis, hangover, irregular periods, indigestion, obesity	Depression, lack of energy, feelings of imbalance and confusion	Avoid if pregnant, taking contraceptive pill, are epileptic, or have sensitive skin.	Middle
FRANKINCENSE (regulating)	General aches and pains, coughs, mature or problem skin, scarring, burns, skin blemishes	Confusion, lack of confidence, jitteriness, panic attacks, stress disorders	There are no specific safety precautions.	Base
GINGER (stimulating)	Rheumatism, constipation, diarrhea, indigestion, poor circulation	Low sex drive	Use in low dilution. Avoid UV light. Avoid if you have sensitive skin.	Top
JASMINE (stimulant)	Painful periods, dysentery, hepatitis, swollen breasts, breast-feeding problems	Lethargy, depression, anxiety	Avoid if pregnant or if you have kidney problems.	Middle

ESSENTIAL OIL	PROBLEMS TREATED	EMOTIONS TREATED	SAFETY PRECAUTIONS	NOTE
JUNIPER (stimulant)	Cellulitis, cystitis, rheumatic pains, skin problems, swelling	Stress-related disorders, panic attacks, confusion	Avoid if pregnant or if you have kidney problems.	Middle
LAVENDER (sedating)	Acne and other skin problems, burns, colic, migraine, insect bites	Fear, insomnia, insecurity, stress-related disorders	There are no specific safety precautions.	Middle
LEMON (stimulant)	Cellulitis, chest infections, colds, flu, congestion, nausea, warts	Depression, anxiety, stress-related disorders	Avoid if pregnant. Avoid exposure to ultraviolet light.	Top
LEMONGRASS (stimulant)	General aches and pains, appetite loss, indigestion and related disorders, insect bites, infections	Anxiety, depression, lack of energy, stress	Avoid or test first if you have sensitive skin.	Top
MANDARIN (sedating)	Acne and oily skin, digestive problems, hiccups	Insomnia, nervous tension, anxiety	Avoid exposure to ultraviolet light.	Middle
MARJORAM (sedating)	Asthma, colds, migraine, muscle spasm, rheumatic pains	Anxiety, hyperactivity, panic attacks, nervousness	Avoid if pregnant. Use in low dilutions (1 percent).	Middle
NEROLI (sedating)	Stretch marks and other skin problems, broken veins, diarrhea, jitteriness	Anxiety, hysteria, insomnia, panic, shock, stress	Avoid exposure to ultraviolet light.	Base
ORANGE (uplifting)	Heartburn, indigestion, colic, constipation	Depression, confusion, panic, stress	Avoid exposure to ultraviolet light.	Base
PATCHOULI (uplifting)	Cellulitis, hemorrhoids, varicose veins, acne, eczema and other skin conditions, scars	Depression, exhaustion, low sex drive	Avoid or use low dilution if prone to headaches.	Base
ROSE (regulating)	Period problems, PMS, skin disorders, eczema, asthma, rheumatism	Depression, anxiety, low sex drive, fatigue, insomnia	Carry out a skin test 48 hours beforehand if you have sensitive skin.	Middle
ROSEMARY (stimulating)	Menstrual problems, muscular pain, poor circulation	Depression, mental fatigue	Avoid if you have sensitive skin or are pregnant.	Middle
SAGE (regulating)	Arthritis, rheumatism, menstrual problems, burns, superficial wounds, inflammation	Menopausal and menstrual mood problems, imbalance stress disorders	Avoid if pregnant. Avoid alcohol after use.	Middle
SANDALWOOD (sedating)	Acne, bronchitis, catarrh, cough, cystitis, laryngitis, throat infections	Low sex drive, fear, panic, lack of confidence, anxiety	There are no specific safety precautions.	Base
TEA TREE (stimulant)	Insect bites, burns, athlete's foot, fungal infections, ulcers, spots	Exhaustion, fatigue, lack of energy, imbalance	There are no specific safety precautions.	Top
YLANG YLANG (uplifting)	Acne, skin and hair condition, high blood pressure, palpitations	Anger, frustration, depression, anxiety, low sex drive	Avoid if you have sensitive skin.	Base

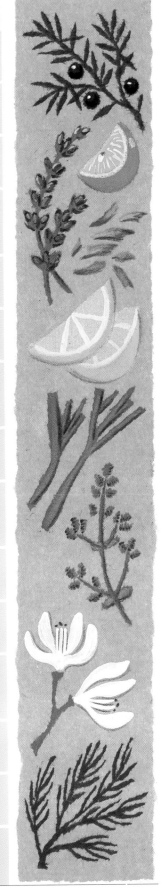

to the skin. Although essential oils are often added to a carrier to enhance the soothing or healing properties of the massage, they are not required.

The most common carrier oil is the nourishing sweet almond oil, known for its soothing and softening properties. Grapeseed oil is also popular and is good for oily skin, although it is not as fine or pure. Sunflower oil is another popular carrier oil; it contains vitamins A, B, D, and E and is relatively inexpensive. It is also good for helping to relieve bronchitis and asthma. The last two oils are neutral in odor and for this reason absorb essential oils well.

Apricot kernel oil, which is both penetrating and rich in minerals, is also commonly used as a carrier oil; it is particularly effective for mature skins.

Certain carrier oils that have special properties are blended with other carriers. For example, avocado oil has many nutrients, including vitamins A, B, and D, but is too thick and must be diluted with another carrier like sweet almond oil—about 1 part avocado to 3 parts sweet almond. It keeps well due to its antioxidant qualities. Sesame oil is another one that is rich in vitamins and can be used to improve lighter oils. It is particularly good for treating psoriasis and eczema.

Jojoba is a wax from a desert plant which, when added to an oil blend, stabilizes the mixture and increases the shelf life. It is anti-inflammatory and balancing.

Wheat-germ oil has powerful antioxidant properties and, when added to other base oils, can help to lengthen their shelf life. It is always good to add 5 to 10 percent of wheat-germ oil to a blend in order to help it maintain potency for a longer period of time.

BUYING AND STORING OILS

Carrier oils can be bought from any reputable aromatherapy supplier or health store; they should be cold-pressed and not contain any additives.

Vegetable oils can go rancid, or oxidize, quickly, especially if they are left open. It is best to buy them in limited quantities so it won't be necessary to store them for long. To prevent oils from going rancid, store them in clean, dark, airtight containers away from sunlight. A cool, dry pantry, for example, is a good place. If you use a carrier oil that has preservative qualities, such as jojoba, your massage oils will generally have a greater shelf life.

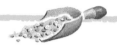

OATMEAL BODY SCRUB

This simple, traditional mixture is used to exfoliate the top layer of dead skin and allow the pores to open and flush out dirt. It will leave your skin feeling refreshed and healthy.

100 g (1¼ cups) coarsely ground oatmeal
100 g (⅓ cup) finely ground sea salt

100 g (½ cup) granulated white sugar

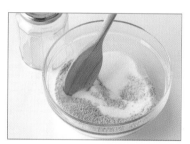

1 *Mix the ingredients together in a large bowl, then transfer the blended mixture to a screw-top jar.*

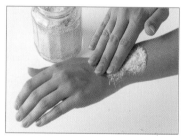

2 *Dampen skin with a sponge or washcloth; pour a small amount of mixture into the palm of your hand and rub into the skin.*

3 *Leave the mixture on for a few minutes, then rinse thoroughly with warm water. It might be helpful to use a washcloth or loofah to remove all traces. Pat your skin dry and apply a moisturizer or body lotion.*

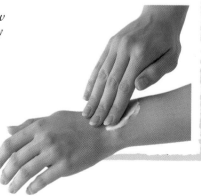

DID YOU KNOW?
Sweet and heady jasmine is reputed to be an aphrodisiac. When the grand duke of Tuscany acquired a plant from India in the 16th century, he forbade anyone to take a cutting. As the story goes, however, his gardener stole a posy of jasmine for his beloved, and won over by its beauty and scent, she planted the cuttings and sold them until she had enough money to wed the poor gardener.

Index

ACKNOWLEDGMENTS

Carroll & Brown Limited
would like to thank
Maddalena Bastianelli
Roselyn Journeaux
Robert St John

Brain Gym
  Edu-K UK consultant
  12 Golders Rise
  London NW4 2HR

British School of Osteopathy
  1–4 Suffolk Street
  London SW1Y 4HG
  tel (0171) 930 9254

International Institute of Reflexology
  32 Priory Road
  Portbury
  Bristol BS20 9TH
  tel/fax (01275) 373359

Editorial assistance
Denise Alexander
Nadia Silver

Design assistance
Simon Daley

DTP design
Elisa Merino

Photographic assistant
Mark Langridge

Picture research
Sandra Schneider

Photograph sources
8 (Top) Vatican Museums and Galleries, Vatican City, Italy/ Bridgeman Art Library, London
10 (Top) Wellcome Institute Library, London
12 (Top) The Kobal Collection
16 (Left) Ancient Art and Architecture Collection (Middle) Wellcome Institute Library, London (Right) Ancient Art and Architecture Collection
17 (Left) Agnew & Sons, London/ The Bridgeman Art Library, London (Middle) Wellcome Institute Library, London (Right) The British Library
18 (Left) Ancient Art and Architecture Collection (Middle) Dr Jeremy Burgess/Science Photo Library (Right) Mary Evans Picture Library
19 (Top) Wellcome Institute Library, London (Left) AKG London (Middle) Mary Evans Picture Library (Right) Pictorial Press
21 CNRI/Science Photo Library
31 E.T.Archive
36 (Top) Private Collection/The Bridgeman Art Library, London (Bottom) Mary Evans Picture Library

40 Tony Stone Images
43 Tony Stone Images
51 Good Housekeeping/Alex James
52 Jules Selmes
54 Jules Selmes
62 Mary Evans Picture Library
64 British School of Osteopathy
65 Tony Stone Images
76 Ron Thompson
84 International Institute of Reflexology
96 G. Hadjo/Science Photo Library
100 Images Colour Library

Illustrators
John Batten
Rosamund Fowler
John Geary
Sandy Hill
Frances Lloyd
Evie Loizides
Joanna Venus
Paul Williams

Hair and make-up
Bettina Graham
Kim Menzies

Index
Jennifer Mussett